The How to Eat for CKD Method
The Core Method

The How to Eat for CKD Method, The Core Method

The Highly Adaptable Method to Successfully Make those Dietary Changes for a Lifetime of Kidney-Friendly Eating. Part Two of the Two-part Method.

Linda Blaylock

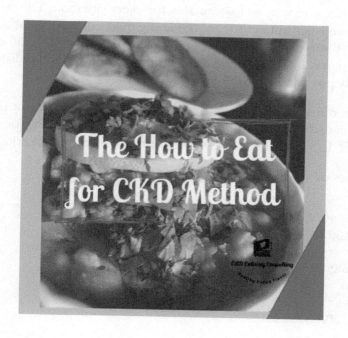

CKD Culinary Consulting
2023

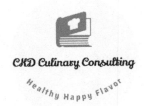

CKD Culinary Consulting

Healthy Happy Flavor

DEDICATION

This book is dedicated to kidney disease warriors everywhere.
The CKD community is my inspiration and reason for doing what I do.

Welcome!

I am so happy you are continuing and taking the steps to learn how to make those dietary changes. This is part two of the method program. Here you will have access to the core method of the program that elevates your kidney diet, shows you how to make those dietary changes, and assures they fit your specific dietary needs. This program is designed to fully arm you with everything you need, to make things as easy as possible, and to give you your monetary investment's worth!

If you purchased my first book, which laid the foundation and supplied you with all the basic information you will need, then, you already know my name is Linda, and I am a chef, a certified nutritionist, a kidney health coach, as well as a caregiver to my husband who has stage three kidney disease.
I will spare you my story as I assume you've read it.

So, as our reigning round one champion, what should you expect this time around?

You will be given a lot of information and it may seem overwhelming at times, but I promise it gets easier and easier with the continued use of the steps and information.

This program will require your full commitment and dedication to succeed. Please do not jump ahead in the modules as they build on top of each other.
There is information you will need to know from one module to the next to implement this correctly.

You will also need the reference materials from the previous book.
Please take the time you need to work through the units. Some are quick, some are more involved.

You are ready to dive straight into round two, and start on the journey that is going to change your life when it comes to CKD eating.
Again, congratulations on taking this next step. I am so excited for you!

So, why don't we just get you started. The sooner, the better, for your kidneys (and your sanity!).

Linda

Welcome Back, Round 1 Champion!

The mission of CKD Culinary Consulting is to help, support, and empower kidney disease patients with the tools to execute dietary success within their restrictions and preferences.

Here we are...

Building off the foundational information in book one, this continues with an easy to follow, step-by-step method, guiding patients on how to make the necessary dietary changes. This supplies the vital processes and information to finally make the transition into kidney-friendly eating simple, easy, effective, and enjoyable for life.

The core method supplies complete information to ease stress and end the confusion of the current kidney diet. It moves patients from struggling to succeeding. The complete process is highly adaptable, cannot be found anywhere else. Join the many others that have breathed a sigh of relief and are living their best CKD lives right now.

Medical Disclaimer

For informational purposes only.

With purchase of this book, or acceptance of by gift, or use of any information with, you accept and agree that:

This work is offered with the understanding that CKD Culinary Consulting, LLC is not rendering medical, legal, or other professional advice or services. Seek professional services if needed. No guarantee to health or the slowing or halting of kidney disease is expressed.

Although every effort is made to ensure the accuracy of information shared, the information may inadvertently contain inaccuracies or typographical errors. You agree that CKD Culinary Consulting, LLC. is not responsible for the views, opinions, or accuracy of facts referenced, or of those of any other individual or company affiliated with our business in any way. Because scientific, technology, and business practices are constantly evolving, you agree that **CKD Culinary Consulting, LLC. is not responsible for the accuracy, or for any errors or omissions that may occur.**

All recipes supplied, or any nutritional information given in any capacity is not guaranteed for accuracy. All information is obtained using reputable sources. All recipes are calculated using the NB20 program which is linked to the USDA. Recipes are not lab tested; therefore, accuracy is not guaranteed.

Any mistypes, inaccuracies, or omissions are not intentional and can be brought to our attention to remedy. We do our best to supply information as close to accurate as possible however, many times nutritional data may not be available and amounts are estimated based on the next best food or product, or on the base ingredients used. A statement will often accompany when this has occurred. We make every attempt to capture accurate information and will often contact the company requesting that information. As new food testing comes forward, this can alter the information we had previously supplied. When it is found or brought to our attention, information will be updated to the best of our ability.

No guarantees may be created or extended by use of the materials within. Advice, strategies, suggestions, menus, methods, information, recipes, etc., may not be suitable for every situation.

The recipes and suggestions within are based on Stage 3 kidney disease, as this is the largest known group. However, whenever possible, suggestions are listed to adjust for other stages or dietary preferences. There is no guarantee that those adjustment suggestions will fit your needs.

CKD Culinary Consulting offers no guarantee or undertaking and makes no representation of any kind that the program or products will meet Your requirements, achieve any intended results, be compatible or work with any other dietary needs.

This information is for home use only. This is shared information based on experiences.

No liability is assumed by CKD Culinary Consulting, LLC for this information, for any misuse, misdirection, or situations arising from what you do with this information.

Now that we have that out of the way, let's get you going!!

Table Of Contents

WELCOME BACK, ROUND ONE CHAMP

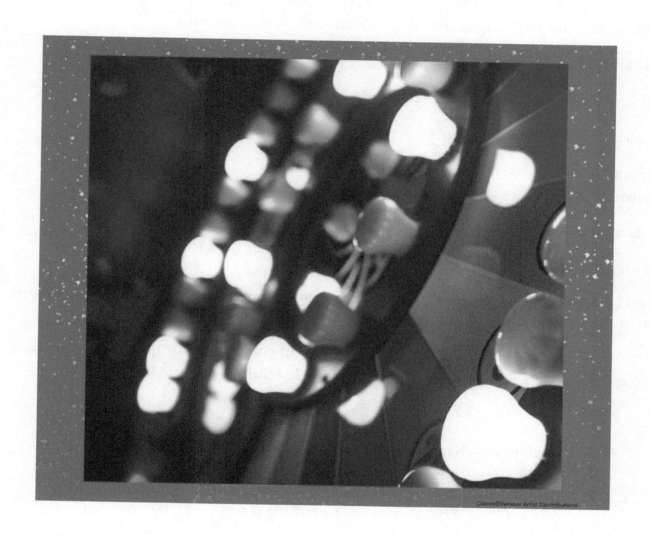

LET'S MAKE SURE YOU HAVE THIS INFORMATION UP FRONT

It is truly an honor to help you on this continued journey.

Now, if you remember from book one, you can schedule assistance calls for issues you need clarification on.

I've been in your shoes; I know how some of the information in this book can seem overwhelming or a bit confusing.

Maybe you just have a question or want clarification on something.

 I can help.

To ensure you receive the help you need, you can schedule an assistance call!

Calls are 30 minutes via zoom®.

If you would like to schedule one, head on over here: **https://www.howtoeatforckd.com/**

Click the button for assistance calls and schedule it for your earliest convenience.

There is a reasonable charge for the calls.

Fees are not refundable for any reason. If you cannot make it, do not show up, forget, etc. You forfeit the fee as an administrative inconvenience charge.

If you would like to join the accompanying support community for this book, please go here: **https://www.facebook.com/groups/h2e4ckdpro**

As you move to the chapters, take note that they are not 1, 2, 3… but instead, are a continuation from book one. 5, 6, 7…

Now that the reminders are done, jump on in!

More Helpful Information

Let's start out in the same manner as book one by touching on some common issues with CKD. First up, let's talk about a big one, the annoying one... Pruritis.

Pruritis (Itching)

Crazy annoying and frustrating too. It is quite common with kidney disease, especially end-stage or when on dialysis.

It can sometimes cause red or different colored patches of skin and is often on the arms, head, abdomen, or back, but it can be almost anywhere and everywhere.

Currently, **the cause** is not known. There are some ideas and theories within the medical community such as:

- Long-term inflammation and/or swelling.
- Dry skin which is common for those on dialysis due to the loss of sweat glands
- High phosphorus levels
- Hyperparathyroidism
- High levels of aluminum and magnesium
- Not attending all dialysis appointments (leading to mineral build ups)

Symptoms aren't always the same for everyone.
- For some, the itching may be constant, for others it may be reoccurring or cyclic
- Can feel differently, some feel itchy, or crawly, or prickly
- Scratching does not relive the feelings
- Skin can become dry, raw, and have an uneven skin tone
- Sleep disturbances are common
- Hot whether can aggravate it
- Stress can also contribute
- No matter how it feels, it's freaking annoying to deal with!

Treatment options can be discussed with your doctor. Currently, these are the best options:
- Attend all dialysis appointments to avoid excessive mineral build ups
- Lotions may help
- Switch soaps and laundry detergents to those made for sensitive skin
- When bathing or showering, avoid hot water, try cool or lukewarm
- Use a humidifier in your home, have a second smaller one in the bedroom as you sleep
- Avoid scratching which can make it worse, can damage the skin, and lead to infections
  - If you've ever watched the TV show friends, I think of the episode where Pheobe had oven mitts duct taped to her hands. I guess you could give that a try.

- Try rubbing or applying a cold, wet cloth to irritating patches
- Try an oatmeal bath or applying anti-itching creams (thank goodness oatmeal isn't super expensive!)
- Try skin sensitizing items that you can gently drag or brush over your skin which will not remove or damage your skin but allows the sensation to aid in relief. Ya know, there's probably a word for that but, I chose to use the long, comforting sounding explanation.
- Reduce calcium, phosphorus, magnesium, and aluminum by following a kidney friendly diet (yep, me again. Here to help)
- Have your parathyroid hormones tested and talk with your doctor
- Antihistamines
- Ask your doctor about medication options. The FDA has approved a drug that can be administered during hemodialysis (not available for peritoneal)

Dealing with pruritis daily can take a toll.
It can lead to anxiety, depression, or other mental health issues. Keep that in mind and know you are living with the effects of your disease. Know it is not your fault, and never apologize or feel ashamed.
And if anyone asks why you have an entire drawer full of oven mitts and duct tape, you could choose to tell them it's your condition, or not. Ha!
(American Kidney Fund, n.d.)

Polycystic Kidney Disease (PKD)

This is a genetic disease, meaning there's a mutation in your genes that causes cysts to grow inside the kidneys. There can be thousands of fluid-filled cysts which can damage the kidneys and make your kidneys larger than normal. Some cysts can become excessively large.
(American Kidney Fund, n.d.)

There are two types of **PKD**:

ADPKD (autosomal dominant)
- This can also affect other organs, especially the liver.
- About half of the people with this will have kidney failure by age 70. Let's hope you're in the half that doesn't have that happen.
- Symptoms often start between ages 30 and 50. Ya probably think it's aging but, it may not be. Get checked!
- Is the most common type, and is also called adult PKD
- This genetic change can happen on its own, without having received this awful gift from your parents. This is rare. But since it can happen, don't run off and start yelling at your parents.
- Genes are passed from parents to children. This is not a gift we are thankful for.
  - If one parent has the ADPKD gene, you have a 50% chance of being born with it
  - If both parents have it, your chances of being born with it increase to 75%
  - I like to look at that as 50% and 25% chance, respectively, of not being born with it

- **Symptoms**
  - Headaches
  - High blood pressure
  - Pain in your back or sides
  - Kidney stones
  - Urinary tract infections

- **Treatment**
  - Talk to your doctor about medications
  - Follow a kidney friendly diet (which I am helping you with!)
  - Get active. Wiggle in your chair, get up and dance, go for a walk…
  - As always, stop those "bad" habits like excessive alcohol and smoking

ARPKD (autosomal recessive)
- Can be severe and deadly for newborns
- More than half of babies born with this will have kidney failure by mid-teens to early twenties
- This too can also affect other organs, again, especially the liver
- This is much less common and also called infantile PKD

- A genetic disease that disrupts the normal development of the liver and kidneys

- **Symptoms** or other health issues
    - Underdeveloped lungs
    - High blood pressure
    - Liver problems
    - Internal bleeding
    - Excessive thirst and urination
    - Enlarged kidneys
    - Swollen abdomen
    - Feeding problems and stunted growth
    - Kidney disease and failure

- **Treatment**
    - Medication
    - Ventilator, if needed
    - Surgery, if needed
    - Dialysis
    - Transplant

Sadly, depending on the severity, it can be fatal. Common ages of death are age 5, mid-teens, and early 20's. Celebrate them while you have them.
(National Institute of Health, n.d.)

Kidney Stones

We all know that our kidneys filter waste from our blood. When we aren't drinking enough or our body isn't producing enough urine, crystals form inside the kidneys.

Other waste that is being filtered will glob on to the crystals and form a stone (or stones), which can range in size from teeny tiny to super large, think golf ball.

Anyone can get these but some people, like men, get them more often.

So, are you at risk?
- Not drinking enough fluids
- Consuming large amounts of protein
- Eating a lot of sugar or salt
- Family history or you've had them previously
- Medications like diuretics
- If you consume a lot of calcium-based medications or antacids
- If you are overweight or have other health issues like PKD
    - Especially issues that affect the levels of cystines, oxalates, uric acid, or calcium in your body

How do you know if you have them?
- Feeling nauseated or throwing up
- Pain in you lower abdomen or back
- Cloudy, bloody, or stinky urine,
- Painful urination

Treatment
- There are different treatments, depending on some factors like the size and type of the stone. Stones can be made of different things, so treatment varies.
- Passing stones, as we've all heard, is painful and if the stones are too large to pass, surgery is needed.
- Lithotripsy is the treatment we hope for. This uses shock waves to break the stone into small pieces that you can hopefully pass without unbearable pain.
- There's a procedure that is going to make you squirm a bit. Ready? Ureteroscopy.
    - Lemme break this down for you…
        - Ureter: the long tubes that take the urine from the kidneys, all the way out of your body.
        - Scopy: is the medical term for going on in there and looking.
        - The O that was not included in those two broken up sections, let's just say it stands for **Oh** Sh….
            - Yep, they are going to use a tool to go on up in there and take out the stone.
            - You okay? Sitting alright?

Moving on…

So, how do you keep them at bay?

Essentially, do the opposite of the risky behaviors listed above.

- Drink enough fluids
- Limit protein, sugar, and salt
- Stop popping the calcium meds or those antiacids
- Ya can't really stop the genetics (yet), but you can change your diet to lower those oxalates, cystines, etc.

Remember I mentioned earlier that there are different types of stones?

There are four.

Calcium is the most common. If someone is monitoring their oxalates, this is probably why. This is a good reason to drink your fluids.

Uric are common. High levels of purines encourage your body to produce high levels of uric acid. This is one that you will not thank your parents or grandparents for passing on to you. It's also the reason to avoid that tasty seafood.

Struvite is not as common. If you are part of the frequent UTI (urinary tract infection) club, these are the ones you are probably dealing with. The bacterium from that infection is the culprit.

Cystine is far less common. These are caused by a rare condition called cystinuria that you got handed down to you from somewhere in the family. Your body leaks cystines into your urine where they all get together and form a stone. Ahh…. Family. Sadly, like a bad relative that won't leave, these guys will stay in your kidneys, bladder, or whatever spot they choose to pitch a tent within your urinary tract. This is an incurable condition.

(American Kidney Fund, 2022)

High Blood Pressure

Holds the number two title for the cause of kidney disease.

Your kidneys are one of the key players in keeping your blood pressure in check. When your kidneys aren't happy, they can't do the job.

Think of those days, probably in your late 20's when you were out the night before partying pretty hard and on Friday came in but really didn't do much work cos you felt like he!!.

Now imagine if you were being forced to do hard labor. No way you are going to keep up, right?

So, when your kidneys can't keep up, a nasty little cycle happens.

Your blood pressure is rampaging, your kidneys become damaged, your blood pressure is still wreaking havoc, and in turn your kidneys are taking the brunt of it, then your heart starts to get involved in this little spat, and it all gets to be a crazy mess.

Top priority, get that blood pressure under control, maybe even have it apologize too. It's been running amuck, causing your blood vessels to constrict and narrow, which not only harmed the kidneys, but the rest of your body as well.

I don't feel I need to go into all the statistics, treatments, symptoms, etc. cos most everyone already knows this information.

So, I will cover the one thing that everyone forgets, systolic and diastolic.

The **TOP** number is systolic and is the pressure (think squeezing) that occurs when your heart beats and is pushing the blood through your blood vessels.

The **BOTTOM** number is diastolic and is the pressure that occurs as the blood vessels relax between heartbeats (think relax and refill).

To help remember this, think of squeezing something, S for squeeze and systolic.

Then think of dropping the item you squeezed while you sigh; it drops to the ground, D for drop and diastolic (bottom number) as you release a relaxing breath.

You're welcome.

Diabetes

Here we have the reining champ, the number one cause of CKD.

In fact, one in three adults that have diabetes also have kidney disease. Basically, one third.

Both types, 1 and 2 can cause kidney disease.

The big question I had was, how does diabetes cause kidney disease? I mean, I get the high blood pressure thing, but not everyone who has diabetes has high blood pressure. So…

Here's the answer:

The continued high blood sugar damages blood vessels and those tiny little nephrons in the kidneys. This is why many people with diabetes end up with high blood pressure.

Now you know! Now you see the connection. Now you see the terrible little cycle, right?

Much like with high blood pressure, I am not going to go into much details cos it is already widely known information.

Let's cover this little gem cos somebody is dealing with this and hopefully this alerts them to it!

PREdiabetes.

This is where blood sugar levels are consistently elevated but not high enough to warrant the dreaded type 2 diagnosis. This is your chance to get things under control now!

Sadly, most people aren't aware they are prediabetic.

Symptoms

- Thirsty
- Frequent urination
- Fatigue
- Blurred vision
- Increased hunger
- Numbness or tingling feet and hands
- Weight loss (this may excite some people but, really, it's a warning sign!)
- Fasting blood sugar level between 100 to 125 milligram/dL
- An A1C test between 5.7% and 6.4%

If any of these things are going on for you or someone you love, get them checked.

Okay, the rest is common knowledge, especially if you have diabetes.

Stop smoking, exercise, lose weight, drop carbs, yadda, yadda…

Let's move on…

Anemia

Generally, it means your hemoglobin (red blood cells) is less than 12.0 - 13.0 g/dL.
When GFR drops below 60, anemia can start to develop.
Yep, another nasty loop. As the GFR drops, the chances of developing or worsening anemia go up, which further damages the kidneys, around, and around.

Anemia is common and sadly leads to poor outcomes. I don't want to say it, I know you don't want to hear it, especially if this is you. But, yes, death.

60% of those not on dialysis are dealing with anemia.
Now, the sad part is, the medical community is struggling to treat this. The best option is to improve renal function and increase red blood cell production. To do so, diet (um, hi again) is key, playing a significant role. Incorporating stimulating agents to get your body producing those red blood cells, and iron supplementation are next.
Along with this, the deficiency of vitamins that Iron is best friends with can make things much worse. Yet another reason to make sure your diet is nutritionally maximized within your limitations!

I hate to add another depressing fact here but, most patients do not respond to the stimulating agents, and this (continued hemoglobin deficiency) often results in death from a cardiovascular event (think heart attack and heart failure).
Always follow up with your doctor regarding iron supplements. There are different kinds of iron and different doses. The root cause plays a factor as well.
(Shaikh H, 2023)

Symptoms

- Shortness of breath
- Fatigue and/or weakness
- Dizzy
- Headaches
- Cannot concentrate
- Rapid heartbeat
- Chest pains
- Severe anemia can cause heart failure

Here's the foods that can help. You will need to make sure you are keeping within your nutritional window when consuming. Make sure to balance these out but use them each day, if possible.

Red meat (the redder, the better), poultry, pork, seafood, beans, dark leafy greens (usually high in potassium!), dried fruit (also high in potassium!), Iron-fortified foods, peas, broccoli, sweet potatoes, green beans, whole wheat products, whole grain products, bran products, corn meal, strawberries, watermelon, tofu, kidney beans, garbanzo (chickpeas) beans, tomatoes, lentils, maple syrup, molasses, eggs, nuts.
https://www.healthdirect.gov.au/foods-high-in-iron

Let's keep going. I am afraid it won't get any better in the next couple pages, but you should know this stuff!

Oxalates

AKA: oxalic acid. An abundance in the body leads to a condition called hyperoxaluria (too much oxalate in your urine). (Cleaveland Clinic, n.d.)

This can lead to health issues such as kidney stones, which in turn, yep… kidney disease.

When the kidneys can't flush the excess oxalates out, they will build up in other areas of the body causing:

- Bone disease
- Anemia
- Heart problems
- Skin problems
- Eye problems
- Growth and development problems in children

This build up is called oxalosis.

What's the symptoms, you ask?

- Blood in the urine
- Unable to urinate, frequent or painful urination
- Urine that is stinky or cloudy
- Fever and/or chills
- Pain on the side of the body or lower back which can become so intense as to cause nausea and/or vomiting

Let's break this down, there are two types.

Primary is a rare genetic disorder (ah, those genetics again). This causes the liver to not produce enough of the enzymes needed to prevent high oxalate levels, or those enzymes are way too lazy and refuse to work.

Secondary is a condition where the gastrointestinal tract is absorbing way too many oxalates, this is common for people with Crohn's disease or Inflammatory bowel disease, disorders where nutrients are not properly absorbed, and for those who've had gastric bypass surgery or intestinal surgery.

So, what do **treatments** look like?

- Medications, of course
- Increasing fluids
- Changing your diet (um… yep. Hi. Again)
    - Dietary changes are not very helpful if you have primary hyperoxaluria, as it is genetics)
- Jump back up to kidney stones, this applies if stones are occurring.
- Consuming calcium rich foods (calcium binds to oxalates, which results in expulsion through stool instead of urine)

So, for those dietary changes, it is suggested to lower your intake of:

- Dairy
- Eggs
- Fish
- Salt
- Sugar

These should be **avoided**:

- ☠ Amaranth
- ☠ Beans and bean products
- ☠ Beets
- ☠ Blackberries
- ☠ Buckwheat
- ☠ Chia seeds
- ☠ Chocolate (right? nooooooooo!!!)
- ☠ Figs
- ☠ Juices (due to the excessive Vitamin C)
- ☠ Kiwi
- ☠ Nuts and nut products
- ☠ Plums
- ☠ Pomegranate
- ☠ Potatoes and potato products
- ☠ Rhubarb

- ☠ Sesame seeds
- ☠ Soy /tofu
- ☠ Spinach
- ☠ Star fruit
- ☠ Strawberries
- ☠ Sweet potatoes
- ☠ Swiss Chard

Your **better** options are:

- ✓ Apples
- ✓ Avocado
- ✓ Blueberries
- ✓ Calcium-rich foods
- ✓ Cauliflower
- ✓ Cherries
- ✓ Coconut
- ✓ Cucumber
- ✓ Grapes
- ✓ Kale
- ✓ Red bell peppers
- ✓ Squash

These are not complete lists.

If you need help, you can head over here: https://oxalate.org/

Soft Foods

This is a thing, a common thing! I get a lot of requests from people either with dental issues, or they recently had dental work done and aren't sure how to handle it.
Lemme help.

The key is to keep nutrition maximized.
Here are lists of your top options that are workable.

- **Grains** can be cooked to make porridge.
  - o BEST OPTIONS Based on potassium and phosphorus amaranth, pearled barley, farro, millet, oat **bran (not oats. If you want oats, stick to 4 ounces per day)**, rice.
- **Beans** can be cooked down (think refried). 1/4 to 1/2 cup per meal, depending on other ingredients.
  - o BEST OPTIONS Based on potassium and phosphorus tofu, canned chickpeas, canned red kidney, canned pinto. 1/4 to 1/2 cup per meal, depending on other ingredients.
- **Pasta** can also be cooked down to a mooshy state and incorporated into a meal.
- **Soft, fresh cheeses** can be incorporated. Limit to 1 ounce per meal.
- **Eggs** are a wonderful option and work in nearly anything. Keep to 2 eggs per meal.
- **Fish** can also be cooked down to soft. 3-4 ounces per meal.
- **Gluten free products** are often softer and crumblier. They may be easier to eat than regular breads, cookies, etc.
- **Dairy products** should be limited to 1 or 2 ounces per meal and stick to the high fat versions.
- **Fruits**: Choose the canned versions, pureed (like applesauce), juices, etc. Make sure you are not exceeding your potassium for the day!

  - o Apple juice (not potassium added)
  - o Applesauce, canned
  - o Apricot nectar, canned
  - o Blackberry juice, canned
  - o Blueberries, canned, frozen, raw
  - o Cranberry sauce, jellied or whole
  - o Cranberry juice
  - o Fruit cocktail, canned
  - o Gooseberries, canned
  - o Grape juice
  - o Guava nectar, canned
  - o Loganberries, frozen, raw
  - o Lychee, canned, raw, frozen
  - o Mango nectar
  - o Mangosteen (a berry, not mango), canned

- o Papaya, canned
- o Papaya nectar, canned
- o Peach nectar, canned
- o Peaches, canned, frozen
- o Pears, Bosc, raw
- o Pears, Red & Green Anjou, raw
- o Pears, canned, raw, frozen
- o Pear nectar
- o Guanabana (soursop, graviola, guayabano) nectar
- o Strawberries, canned, frozen
- o Watermelon, raw, frozen

- **Vegetables:** Stick to canned or cooked and mashed or pureed. Make sure you do not exceed your potassium for the day!

  - o Beans, green (snap, string, wax), canned, boiled
  - o Cucumber, raw, peeled or unpeeled
  - o Gourds (wax, tinda, ridge, dishcloth, marrow), raw or cooked
  - o Squash, summer, patty pan (scallop), unpeeled or peeled, raw or lightly cooked
  - o Squash, winter , pumpkin, raw or cooked
  - o Gourd (snake), raw or cooked
  - o Peas, green, canned, frozen
  - o Squash, winter (butternut), frozen then cooked

- **Cook 'n Serve Puddings made with whole milk.**
- **J-ello cups**
- **Pea, vegetable, grain, or bean soups blended down.**

Dialysis

I have to say I am flabbergasted by the number of people on dialysis that are being fed an enormous shovel full of sh***y information while in clinic!!

Let's say this right now…
Unless the person you are dealing with is a renal nurse, specialist, doctor, etc. do **NOT** listen to their advice. Some of the stuff people have been told is quite harmful!

If you are working in that field, unless you are a renal specialist, do **NOT give** advice!

Now, please understand that when you enter dialysis, there are a few things to keep in mind.

Within the first 5 years of dialysis, the **survival rate is about 50%**

The FIRST YEAR of dialysis has the **highest mortality rates, about 30%.**

Yes, that means of the 50% survival rate within the first five years, **30%** of them die within the first year. (Bhandari S, Am J Nephrol 2022;53:32–40)

Stop right here and take that in.
I'll wait.

For a trickle of salt on that wound… 90% of those on dialysis, will eventually develop anemia. So, head back to the page and read up.

Depending on the type of dialysis you receive, complications can occur. You can do some research to find out more information. I will give you some brief highlights.

Hemodialysis is done in a clinic, or at home where you are fitted with a permanent opening to connect the needles or tubes in which a machine will filter your blood to remove the waste.
The opening, or access point is created when a surgeon connects two of your blood vessels, creating a fistula which will get stronger and larger to accommodate the treatments, or a plastic tube will be placed between the two blood vessels, this is called a graft. (Mayo Clinic, n.d.)

What you have to look forward to (not!):
- Cardiac arrhythmias (irregular beating)
- Bleeding
- Anemia (low red blood cells)
- Cramps
- Nausea and vomiting
- Headache
- Infections are super common.

- Bone diseases
- Itching
- Low or high blood pressure
- Sleep problems
- Pericarditis (heart membrane inflammation, interfering with hearts ability to pump blood)
- Hyperkalemia (high potassium)
- Hypoproteinemia (low protein)
- Hypophosphatemia (low phosphorus)
- Amyloidosis (joint stiffness and pain)
- Electrolyte imbalances
- Fluid overload
- Mental health issues
- Your diet (most likely) will change. You probably will need to increase your protein and may need to limit your fluids.

Peritoneal: usually done at home, 3-5 times per day. A cleansing fluid flows through a tube into your abdomen where the lining of your abdomen, the peritoneum, acts like a filter to remove the waste from your blood. At some point, you must drain that fluid from your abdomen and discard it.

More crap to not be happy about:
- Infections
- Weight gain (I know that stopped some of you in your tracks. Ha!)
- Hernias
- Ineffective
- Avoidance of certain medications
- Avoiding baths, hot tubs, swimming in anything other than a chlorinated pool
- Your diet (most likely) will change. You may need to increase your potassium and sodium and may need to increase your fluids.
- It's also likely that people using peritoneal dialysis will eventually have a decline in kidney function that requires hemodialysis or a kidney transplant. (Mayo Clinic, n.d.)

And so, this ends our dialysis lesson for today.

eGFR Explained

There's a lot that goes into the creation of this number that everyone relies so heavily on.

Estimated glomerular filtration rate. This is a test to measure your level of kidney function to determine your stage.

In book one, we covered the numbers and stages. Here we are talking more about the test.

It is calculated using a formula and is based on the results of your blood creatinine test, your age, body size, gender, and ethnicity.

Here's the catch! If you are under 18, muscular, overweight, or pregnant, this can make the eGFR less accurate.

Now, there have been updates to the equation to remove ethnicity. At the time of this printing, the new CKD-EPI 2021 equation is in effect.

This new formula removes race and the determination of a GFR may be based on a few additional equations.

For reference:

- eGFR$_{cr}$ (calculated using only creatinine)

- eGFR$_{cr-cys}$ (calculated using both creatinine and cystatin C)

- eGFR$_{cys}$ (calculated using only cystatin C)

If you want more info on these babies, look 'em up. For now, I won't get into all of it. This is for informational purposes and to help you learn how to satisfy your curiosity.

What this comes down to is: for those who were diagnosed in the earlier stages of CKD (stage 1 or 2), and especially for Blacks, this may alter the diagnosis. Meaning, if you were diagnosed in one of the earlier stages, you may get bumped out or up! So, if you were diagnosed with stage one, you may not have a CKD diagnosis any longer. If you were diagnosed in stage two, you may be in stage one. Yay! (National Kidney Foundation, n.d.)

We covered creatinine in book one. Your creatinine numbers can change depending on things like dietary changes, exercise changes, and decreased fluid consumption, remember?

If you are unsure of your stage, and have your lab numbers, here's a handy calculator to help you:

https://www.kidney.org/professionals/kdoqi/gfr_calculator

Kidney Kitchen®

Let me start by saying that a portion of my proceeds are given back to American Kidney Fund®. They do an amazing job helping the kidney community in so many incredible ways.

I love being a part of that through my regular donations and the availability of my recipes on their Kidney Kitchen® site.

They do a great job cycling through recipes, depending on the season, so you always have some wonderful options at just the right time.

I am tossing this recommendation in here so as you work through this method, you can use their site as a resource.

Nope, not getting paid to recommend them.
As mentioned, in the past, I was a culinary consultant for them, and the amazing experiences I had, and the fantastic people I worked with, earned my loyalty.

I was able to see behind the scenes of the company and realize how completely genuine they are at helping the CKD community. Their dedication is far beyond any others.
They put people first, and never place money as their priority.

So, please feel free to check out their site: https://kitchen.kidneyfund.org/
And help to support them.

If you are in a spot, look them up, they can help!

5

I'll Take the First Category: It's All Math

Nutrient Calculations

This lesson, we are walking you through how to calculate nutrients.

Believe me, when you must adjust recipes, you want this info! My brain always, always, always shuts down if it even sniffs the possibility of doing math.

Not kidding. It runs away from numbers, and I forget my own birthday, which is a single freaking digit!!

Thank God I was blessed with a human calculator for a hubby. Really, math league in high school. anyways...

You are using Target's Market Pantry® brand, less sodium soy sauce as an example.

Read through the sheet, walk through it a few times, and then grab an item in your pantry and run through some calculations until you feel comfortable with this.

Ready? Set? Go!

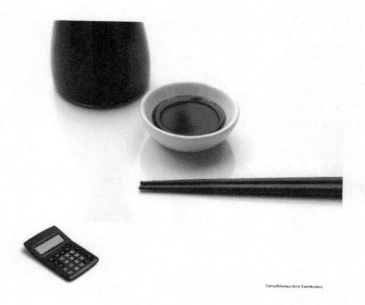

Canva©Various Artist Contributions

How to Calculate the Amount of a Nutrient

TO FIGURE OUT HOW MUCH YOU WILL BE ADDING INTO YOUR FULL RECIPE

- Locate the nutrient amount on the label.
  - o The label for Target's Market Pantry® says that 1 tablespoon of their less sodium soy sauce contains 480 milligrams of sodium. Your recipe calls for 2 tablespoons.
    - Take the 480 (amount per tablespoon) x 2 (number of tablespoons called for in the recipe) = 960 milligrams of sodium that will be added to your full recipe just from the soy sauce.

TO FIGURE OUT HOW MUCH PER SERVING

- Now we need to know how much sodium each serving will have. Your recipe serves 4.
  - o Take the 960 (total amount added to your recipe from the calculation above) and divide by 4 (the number of servings the recipe makes) = 240 milligrams per serving. So, each person will consume 240 milligrams of sodium just from the soy sauce that was used.

FOR TEASPOONS

- If you use teaspoons, let's calculate that out.
  - o The serving size listed on the label says 1 tablespoon and we only want to use 2 teaspoons.
    - Take the 480 (amount per tablespoon in the soy sauce) and divide by 3 (the number of teaspoons in one tablespoon) = 160 milligrams. So, we now know that there are 160 milligrams of sodium per teaspoon.
    - We are using 2 teaspoons in our recipe so take the 160 and multiply by 2 = 320 milligrams of sodium that will go into your recipe.
    - Now continue to divide by the 4 servings. 320 / 4 = 80 milligrams of sodium per serving just from the soy sauce used.

There are other ways to calculate this out that would be quicker, but many people are confused by fractions, percents, and decimals so I simplified it. I think the extra step is worth it.

Also, if you needed to calculate 5 teaspoons, this method is easier.

In this case you would calculate the amount per teaspoon, as done above, then you would multiply it by 5 (the number of teaspoons needed).

You can do this with any nutrient listed on the label.

Conversion Calculations

This lesson will walk you through some obstacles when calculating a recipe using the USDA database. We will also be finishing your list of substitutes.

Let's do this…

First, there will be recipes that you love or come across that you really want to use or try that don't have nutrition listed.

You want a general idea of the nutritional amounts AND you will need to be able to calculate the adjustments that you will most likely have to make.

Second, when you are calculating said recipe, it often happens that the amount listed in the recipe will not be listed as a size option in the USDA. This will help you get around that also.

Two birds, one stone here!

Under 100 grams

So, if the recipe calls for an amount **not** given as an option in the USDA, OR if the recipe you have been calculating needs an adjustment to an ingredient to fit into your restrictions or adaptations, you can easily handle this.

Walk through the steps and calculations on the next sheet, using apricots as an example, to understand how to adjust the amount.

Now, it may happen that after you've adjusted, the nutrition still doesn't work for you, look to reduce the next high potassium item, or make a swap for a lower potassium item.
This is the process you work through with any nutrient that is falling out of line.

Over 100 grams

When you are adjusting, sometimes the amount you are trying to calculate exceeds the default setting in the USDA of 100g.

Here is how you handle this. Work through the sheet, using pastry flour as an example, to understand the process.

You now know and have the resources telling you step-by-step how to reduce amounts and how to calculate those ingredients exceeding 100g.

I know your brain probably hurts right now but hang in there. It gets easier the more you work with this, and you will.

And don't worry, you now have the step-by-step instructions to always come back to and walk you through. Yep, you know it, I still use mine every time!

Conversion Calculations Under 100 grams

There will be times when you need to know the amount of a nutrient (most often, phosphorus), and the information is not available in the serving size or amount you need. Here is where life says, yes! You needed that math class.

Let's use dried apricots as an example.

- Your recipe calls for 1/3 cup of dried apricots, but the USDA only offers 1 cup, 100 grams, or 1 half.
    - To find the amount of phosphorus in 1/3 cup we will first convert it to grams. (We are converting to grams because the USDA will always have a listing of 100 grams)
        - First thing to do is ask Google "how many grams is 1/3 cup of dried apricots" (thank goodness for Google!). Alternately, you can weigh them out yourself.
        - The results show that 1 cup = 190 grams.
        - We need to bring that down to 1/3 cup. So, take the 190 grams and multiply by .33 (the decimal for 1/3 cup)
            - 190 x .33 = 62.7
        - We now know that 1/3 cup of dried apricots is 62.7 (round up to 63) grams.
- In the USDA food database, it shows that 100 grams of dried apricots contain 71 milligrams of phosphorus.
    - We need to know how much is in 63 grams.
        - Take the 71 milligrams and divide it by the 100 grams.
            - 71 / 100 = 0.71
        - Now take the number of grams of our apricots, 63, and multiply it by the 0.71
            - 63 x .71 = 44.73 (round up to 45)
        - We now know that the 1/3 cup in our recipe contains 45 milligrams of phosphorus.
- If you want to know how much per serving, divide the 45 milligrams of phosphorus in our apricots by the number of servings in the recipe (4).
    - 45 / 4 = 11.25
    - We now know that each serving contains 11.25 (or round down to 11) milligrams of phosphorus.

*If you already know the gram amount, start at "take the milligrams and divide it by the 100 grams" in the second step.

If you would like a visual walkthrough, no problem.

Calculations for under 100 grams: https://youtu.be/MNYw2QSGZzc

Conversion Calculations Over 100 grams

If you need to figure out those amounts for ingredients that are over 100 grams (3 1/2 ounces), follow these steps.

Let's use pastry flour as an example.

- Your recipe calls for 4 ounces of flour, but the USDA only offers 100 grams.
  - To find the amount of phosphorus in 4 ounces, we will first convert it to grams.
    - Let's use our math… we know there is 28.35 grams in an ounce. We need to convert the 4 ounces to grams.
    - So, take the 28.35 and multiply it by the 4 ounces. 28.35 x 4 = 113.4. round to 113 for ease.
    - This means that the 4 ounces of flour weighs 113 grams.
  - Now, take the amount of the nutrient, which the USDA says there is 102mg of phosphorus in 100 grams.
    - Take the 102 and divide by the 100 grams. 102 / 100 = 1.02
    - Now multiply the amount listed in the recipe, 113 grams, by the 1.02
      - 113 x 1.02 = 115.668 (round up to 116)
    - We now know that the phosphorus in the 4 ounces of flour is 116 grams.
- If you want to know how much per serving, divide the 116 milligrams of phosphorus by the number of servings in the recipe (12).
  - 116 / 12 = 9.666… round up to 10.
  - We now know that each serving contains 10 milligrams of phosphorus.

If you would like a visual walkthrough, no problem.

Calculations for over 100 grams: https://youtu.be/2LC2fsyw7wg

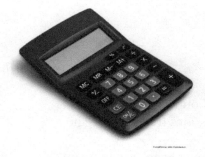

Conversion Calculations to Find 100 grams

Need to know the nutrients in 100 grams exactly?
Here's another situation that may come up.

I found information that said 1 cup of (food item) is 132 grams in weight, and that cup contains 6.7 milligrams of phosphorus.

I had to know the amount for 100 grams so I could move forward with my other calculations.

Here's how you will do this:

- The food item contains 6.7 milligrams of phosphorus per cup.
- I need to know how much phosphorus is in 100 grams.
- Do this:
    - Take the 6.7 milligrams of phosphorus and divide it by the gram amount of 1 cup (132g).
    - **MAKE SURE YOU MOVE THE DECIMAL POINT OVER 2 PLACES!!**
        - **So, instead of 132, it will be 1.32**
            - It looks like this:
                - 6.7 divided by 1.32 = 5.08
- I now know that 100 grams of (food item) contains 5.08 milligrams of phosphorus.

Now you can continue with your other calculations.

BONUS CALCULATION!
*Finding the nutrient amount per **ounce**.*

Most foods are listed as 100g which is about 3 1/2 ounces.

Take the amount of the nutrient, here we will use potassium, and divide it by 3.5.

If veggie x has 230 mg in 100 grams (3 1/2 ounces) then:
230 / 3.5 = 65.714, round up… 66 mg per ounce.

Now, times by the number of ounces you are using. For example, we use 4 ounces in our recipe.
66 milligrams per ounce x 4 ounces in our recipe = 264 milligrams of potassium from this veggie.

We can then divide by the number of servings: 264/4 = 66 mg of potassium in each serving from this veggie.

Nutrient Percentages Calculations

This will walk you through how to calculate out the missing nutrient amounts not listed on the label but are given as a percentage instead.

You know, that little box at the bottom of the nutrition info that always lists a few nutritional items like calcium or iron and then just gives a percentage.

Yeah, who in the heck can look at that and be like, I totally understand what that means and how much that equates to?

Stupid labels.

But, IF we have that percentage, we can figure it out.

It is actually very simple. The key is to have the necessary info to do so.

First, you must have the percentage of the nutrient (usually this will end up being potassium and sometimes phosphorus is listed).

If the percentage is listed, we, **second**, need to have the USDA Daily Recommended Values for said nutrients. Lucky for you, they are listed on the sheet.

Walk through the sheet.

Feel free to grab some other items in your home and calculate those too.

Now…If you do not have the percentage, head on over to the USDA and look up the first ingredient in the list and get an idea of the possible amount from that.

Or you can use your reference sheets (if you have them handy or on your phone) to look up if it is listed in a high, medium, or low category for that nutrient (Potassium or Phosphorus, etc.).

Or, put it back on the shelf. If a product doesn't tell me the potassium, or it lists zero and I know from the ingredient list that that cannot be true, I put it back on the shelf.

If it is something you need and have no other options, use it, and always assume it is higher than what it really is.

Then try emailing the company for the info and hope you hear back in a timely manner.

They won't always have it, especially if they aren't required to test for it or put it on the label.

To me, it is a sign of a good company when they can supply me with that info, and I stick with them if the nutrition is acceptable.

Ok. You are armed and ready!

Calculating Percentages to Find Nutritional Amounts

Sometimes you will find that the information is not available, and you want to figure out how to calculate the amount. This will happen most often with phosphorus since it is not listed on labels.

If the USDA does not have the information (common with name brand items), you can calculate this from the info on the food label (if listed).

- If the package lists the phosphorus (or other ingredients) as a percentage…
  - Multiply the percent listed by the daily value for that nutrient, then divide by 100.
  - Example:
    - Post Grape Nuts Cereal
    - Label says that each serving contains 20% of the Daily Value of phosphorus per serving (1/2 cup).
    - Multiply the 20% by the daily value of phosphorus 1250 (see chart), then, divide by 100.
      - 20% (0.20) x 1250 = 250
    - 250 divided by 100 = 2.5 milligrams of phosphorus per 1/2 cup serving.

Daily Values based on a 2000 calorie diet (USA)

Information current at time of printing. (U.S. Food & Drug Administration, 2022)

Phosphorus 1250 milligrams
Potassium 4700 milligrams
Calcium 1300 milligrams
Iron 18 milligrams
Magnesium 420 milligrams

If the percentage is not listed, find the nutrition info for the first one to three ingredients to give you an idea of the amounts.

BONUS CALCULATIONS!

It happens. Occasionally, a food item will not list 100g. But we need to get it to 100g.

If amount listed is less than 100g, for example, it shows only one size, 1 tablespoon (14g):

Take 100 (grams) and divide by 14g listed = 7.14.
Now, any nutrient you need to know, you will times by the 7.14
If there's 9mg of potassium in the 14g: 9 x 7.14 = 64.26mg of potassium in 100g of that food.

If amount listed is more than 100g, for example, it shows only one size, 1/2 cup (139g):

100g divided by the 139g = 0.719
Now, any nutrient you need to know, you will times by the 0.719
If there's 233mg of potassium in the 139g: 233 x 0.719 = 168mg of potassium in 100g of that food.

Finishing Your List

You had set up your list and have it ready to enter in those nutritional numbers, right?

Here is where we go from there. Start with the ingredient you want to replace. Using okra as an example.

- Ok, I look up OKRA and choose "boiled, without salt". The portions lists 1/2 cup. So, I am going to quickly calculate the numbers for the nutrients we must restrict.

    o 1/4 cup: Potassium is 54 mg, Phosphorus is 13 (rounded up from 12.8), Sodium is 2 (rounded down from 2.4).

    o 1/2 cup: Potassium is 108 mg, Phosphorus is 26 (rounded up from 25.6), Sodium is 5 (rounded up from 4.8).

    o 3/4 cup: here I need to multiply the ½ cup nutrient amount by 1.5 to find the nutritional amounts for ¾ cup. Potassium is 162 mg, Phosphorus is 51 (rounded down from 51.2), Sodium is 7 (rounded down from 7.2).

    o 1 cup: Potassium is 216 mg, Phosphorus is 13 (rounded up from 12.8), Sodium is 10 (rounded up from 9.6).

    o We now know where we nutritionally stand with okra. Now let's find out where we are with our two sub options.

    o

- GREEN BEANS I am choosing the listing "boiled, without salt. They don't offer a steamed or sauteed option, which is what we often do, so I will choose the only other cooked option they have, boiled. 1 cup listing.

    o 1/4 cup: Potassium is 46 mg (rounded up from 45.5), Phosphorus is 9 (rounded down from 9.05), Sodium is 0 (rounded down from 0.3125).

    o 1/2 cup: Potassium is 91 mg, Phosphorus is 18 (rounded down from 18.1), Sodium is 1 (rounded up from 0.625).

    o 3/4 cup: here I need to multiply the 1 cup nutrient amount by 0.75 to find the nutritional amounts for ¾ cup. Potassium is 137 mg (rounded up from 136.5), Phosphorus is 27 (rounded down from 27.15), Sodium is 1 (rounded up from 0.9375).

    o 1 cup: Potassium is 182 mg, Phosphorus is 36 (rounded down from 36.2), Sodium is 1 (rounded down from 1.25).

    o We now know our nutrition for green beans.

- Let's figure out our second sub, BROCCOLI "spears, frozen, cooked" is listed in the medium potassium column. I am choosing the USDA listing for "broccoli, frozen, spears, boiled, without salt" and the 1/2 cup listing.

    o 1/4 cup: Potassium is 83 mg, Phosphorus is 25 (rounded down from 25.3), Sodium is 11 (rounded down from 11.05).

- 1/2 cup: Potassium is 166 mg, Phosphorus is 51 (rounded up from 50.6), Sodium is 22 (rounded down from 22.1).

- 3/4 cup: here I need to multiply the 1/2 cup nutrient amount by 1.5 to find the nutritional amounts for ¾ cup. Potassium is 249 mg, Phosphorus is 76 (rounded up from 75.9), Sodium is 33.

- 1 cup: Potassium is 332 mg, Phosphorus is 101 (rounded down from 101.2), Sodium is 44.

- We now have our info for broccoli.

Follow this example for a clear and easy to use set up:

	Potassium	Phosphorus	Sodium	Include other
Okra				nutrients
1/4 cup	54mg	13mg	2mg	you need
1/2 cup	108mg	26mg	5mg	to track
3/4 cup	162mg	51mg	7mg	
1 cup	216mg	13mg	10mg	
Green Beans				
1/4 cup	46mg	9mg	0mg	
1/2 cup	91mg	18mg	1mg	
3/4 cup	137mg	27mg	1mg	
1 cup	182mg	36mg	154mg	
Broccoli				
1/4 cup	83mg	25mg	11mg	
1/2 cup	166mg	52mg	22mg	
3/4 cup	249mg	75mg	33mg	
1 cup	332mg	101mg	44mg	

We now can look at the nutritional amounts of each to compare and adjust.

We can see that green beans are quite similar, and we can make this swap easily in the same amount as called for in the recipe.

Broccoli is running a bit higher. We will want to reduce the amount we use to better match the nutrition of the original ingredient, okra.

Here, I would reduce the broccoli by half. So, if the original recipe calls for 1/2 cup okra, I will reduce the amount of broccoli and only use 1/4 cup.

We will be using this again and adding in another step. So, hang in there.

If you would like a visual walkthrough, no problem.
You can view it here: https://youtu.be/1xKEJjBWQ5U

Helpful Conversions

Measurement in recipe   =   decimal form for calculations

Fraction	**Decimal**
1/32	0.031
1/16	0.0625
1/8	0.125
1/4	0.25
1/3	0.3333
1/2	0.5
5/8	0.625
2/3	0.667
3/4	0.75
5/6	0.833
7/8	0.875
1	1
1 1/8	1.125
1 1/4	1.25
1 1/3	1.33
1 1/2	1.5
1 5/8	1.625
1 2/3	1.67
1 3/4	1.75
1 5/6	1.83
1 7/8	1.875
2	2

28.35 grams = 1 ounce

If you see a percentage on the label, use this guide.

Percent	Decimal
• 0.5	• 0.005
• 1 (1%)	• 0.01
• 1.5 (1.5%)	• 0.015
• 2 (2%)	• 0.02
• 2.5 (2.5%)	• 0.025
• 3 (3%)	• 0.03
• 3.5 (3.5%)	• 0.035
• 4 (4%)	• 0.04
• 5 (5%)	• 0.05
• 6 (6%)	• 0.06
• 7 (7%)	• 0.07
• 8 (8%)	• 0.08
• 9 (9%)	• 0.09
• 10 (10%)	• 0.1
• 11 (11%)	• 0.11
Etc.	Etc.
• 99	• 0.99
• 100	• 1

Task

I know you may still be working on your subs list, and that is ok. Make darn sure you have it calculated out and ready by the end of the next unit.

Starting in Module 7, you will be using your subs list.

Right now, you can simply focus on this task.

After you have completed this, you will find that calculating your subs list will be a breeze. If you have already completed it, High five! That's awesome.

Are you ready?

Stick to the task sheet **ONLY**.

DO NOT LOOK AT THE RECIPE OR ANSWER SHEET UNTIL YOU ARE DONE!

The task is to calculate the potassium, phosphorus, and sodium in a full recipe.

It might sound scary, but it really isn't. You have a bunch of tools at your disposal, walking you step-by-step. This only seems scary because it is new.

This is giving you a bit of practice on how to calculate a recipe and find the per serving amounts. Repeating the steps helps you absorb the process into your brain.

Keep in mind that the entries in the USDA database that you choose will affect the numbers you get. Remember when we talked about choosing raw, fresh, canned, frozen, etc.?

And when you are calculating, go ahead and Round Up or Down to make it a bit easier to do the math.

When searching, you may need to try different terms and scroll to find the best option and check each tab too.

For example, you won't find seitan, but you will find gluten.

You may look up potato starch, but it is found by searching for flour.

Try several different terms until you find what you need. If the exact item you are looking for isn't listed, use the next closest.

For example, I wanted to look up TVP (texturized vegetable protein). That is not listed in the USDA. But TVP is basically a defatted soy flour product so, I will look up Flour and, in the list, it does have defatted soy flour. I use that listing instead.

When you have finished, look at the answer sheet to see how you did.

If, after you check the answer sheet, you find your numbers are way off, double check the entries you used to calculate each ingredient against the answer sheet, as well as the calculations.

Your numbers may not be the same as what is listed on the answer sheet or recipe. But you should be somewhere near them.

I can't stress this enough; ballpark numbers are fine.

When your numbers are off by 75-100 or more, revisit and recalculate. Often it is simply a selection you make in the database that can alter the numbers greatly.

Remember, there are a lot of foods that can change drastically in nutrition just from cooking them.

Remember to select the item in its state that you add into the recipe. If you are using raw beef and cooking it, then adding more ingredients, select raw.

If you are cooking the meat separately, like for fajitas, and then adding it, select cooked (also watch for the cooking method: broiled, boiled, etc.) always select the option closest to your cooking method.

Sometimes the cooking method used is not listed. Again, choose the one closest to the way you have cooked it.

Once you have completed this, you will have a good understanding of how to calculate recipes and even how to make changes to them.

Grab a pencil and calculator, let's go!

If you would like a visual walkthrough, no problem.

You can view it here: https://youtu.be/r-qnBIXsHmw

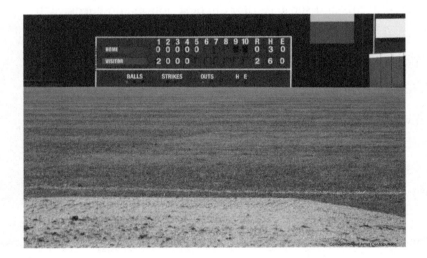

Recipe Info for Task Calculations

CALCULATE THE NURITIONAL AMOUNTS OF POTASSIUM, PHOSPHORUS, AND SODIUM FOR EACH OF THE INGREDIENTS LISTED.

THEN DO A FINAL TALLY

Cheddar Garlic Biscuits

Serving size: 1

Makes: 12

Ingredients:

2 ounces heavy cream

2 tablespoons white vinegar

2 ounces water

90 grams all-purpose flour

30 grams cake flour

1 teaspoon baking powder

1/2 teaspoon garlic powder

1/4 teaspoon baking soda

1 teaspoon caster sugar*

1/2 cup shredded sharp cheddar

1/4 teaspoon Morton's® Kosher coarse salt

4 tablespoons unsalted butter

1/2 tablespoon unsalted butter

1/16 teaspoon garlic powder

1/16 teaspoon Morton's® Kosher coarse salt

*bakers', superfine sugar

Using the USDA Food Database, calculate the Full Recipe and place the totals here:

Potassium:

Phosphorus:

Sodium:

Per Serving (hint = divide by number of servings, 12)

Potassium:

Phosphorus:

Sodium:

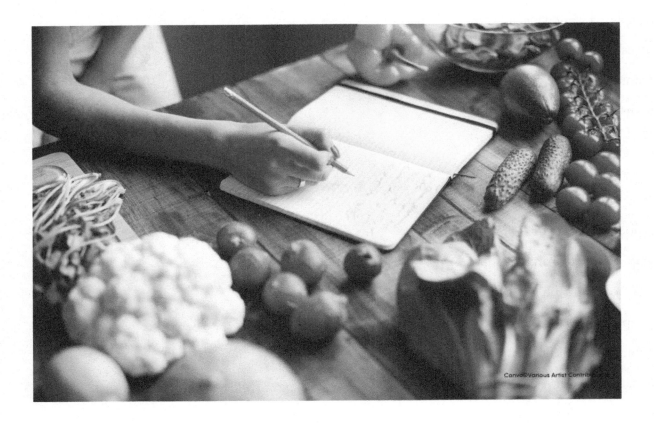

NO PEEKING!

MOD. 5 TASK

Task Answer Sheet

Cheddar Garlic Biscuits
Serving size: 1
Makes: 12

2 ounces heavy cream   Potassium: **57**   Phosphorus: **35**   Sodium: **16**
Survey foods. Cream, heavy. 1oz listing x 2

2 tablespoons white vinegar   Potassium: **1**   Phosphorus: **1**   Sodium: **1**
Legacy foods. Vinegar, distilled. 1T listing x 2

2 ounces water   Potassium: **0**   Phosphorus: **0**   Sodium: **0**
Water contributes nothing

90 grams all-purpose flour   Potassium: **122**   Phosphorus: **104**   Sodium: **4**

Foundation foods. Flour, wheat, all-purpose, enriched, unbleached. 100g listing
Take the phosphorus from the 100g listing (115) and divide it by the 100g.
115 / 100 = 1.15
Take the grams of flour (90) and multiply by the 1.15
90 x 1.15 = 103.5 (round up to 104). Repeat for potassium and sodium.

30 grams cake flour   Potassium: **32**   Phosphorus: **26**   Sodium: **1**

Legacy foods. Wheat flour, white, cake, enriched. 100g listing. Perform the same calculations as for
the 90g flour above.

1 teaspoon baking powder   Potassium: **1**   Phosphorus: **101**   Sodium: **488**

Legacy foods. Leavening agents, baking powder, double acting, sodium aluminum sulfate. 1t listing
Or choose the product you use or the most common on the market.

1/2 teaspoon garlic powder   Potassium: **18**   Phosphorus: **6**   Sodium: **1**
Legacy foods. Spices, garlic powder. 1t
listing. Divided by 2

1/4 teaspoon baking soda   Potassium: **0**   Phosphorus: **0**   Sodium: **630**
Legacy foods. Leavening agents, baking
soda. 1/2t listing. Divided by 2

1 teaspoon caster sugar*   Potassium: **0**   Phosphorus: **0**   Sodium: **0**
This one was tricky as caster/baker's/superfine are not listed. You must use sugars, granulated, under
the Foundation foods. 1tsp listing. Divided by 4

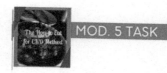

1/2 cup shredded sharp cheddar
Foundation foods. Cheese, cheddar. 1c
listing. Divided by 2

Potassium: 40   Phosphorus: 241   Sodium: 344

1/4 teaspoon Morton's® Kosher coarse salt
Branded foods. Coarse kosher salt. This one is easier to look up the label. Label says 480 per 1/4tsp.
Yes. Sometimes it helps to pull the product up online and use that instead.

Potassium: 0   Phosphorus: 0   Sodium: 480

4 tablespoons unsalted butter
Legacy foods. Butter, without salt.
1T listing. x 4

Potassium: 14   Phosphorus: 14   Sodium: 6

1/2 tablespoon unsalted butter
Legacy foods. Butter, without salt. 1T listing.
Divided by 2

Potassium: 2   Phosphorus: 2   Sodium: 0

1/16 teaspoon garlic powder
Legacy foods. Spices, garlic powder. 1t
listing. Divided by 16

Potassium: 2   Phosphorus: 1   Sodium: 1

1/16 teaspoon Morton's® Kosher coarse
salt

Potassium: 0   Phosphorus: 0   Sodium: 120

Branded foods. Coarse kosher salt. This one is easier to look up the label. Label says 480 per 1/4tsp.
Divided by 4 for the 1/16 t needed. Yes. Sometimes it helps to pull the product up online and use that
instead.

Totals: 289   531   2092

Using the USDA Food Database, calculate the
Full Recipe:
Potassium: 289
Phosphorus: 531
Sodium: 2092

Keep in mind that that the nutrition listed on
the full recipe was calculated using the NB20
program. Your numbers should be
somewhere near those, not necessarily exact.

Per Serving (hint = divide by number of servings, 12)
Potassium: 24
Phosphorus: 44
Sodium: 174

Congratulations!!
I know it is a lot to get through and takes some time.
Once you feel comfortable with this, feel free to use an app or program instead.

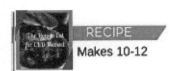

RECIPE
Makes 10-12

Cheddar Garlic Biscuits

Ingredients:
2 ounces heavy cream
2 tablespoons vinegar
About 2 ounces of water
3/4 (90g) cup all-purpose flour
1/4 cup (30g) cake flour (or more all-purpose)
1 teaspoon baking powder
1/2 teaspoon garlic powder
1/4 teaspoon baking soda
1 teaspoon caster (superfine/baker's) sugar
1/2 cup shredded sharp cheddar cheese
1/4 teaspoon Morton's® kosher coarse salt
4 tablespoons melted unsalted butter
1/2 tablespoon more butter, melted for brushing tops
1/16 teaspoon Morton's® kosher coarse salt
1/16 teaspoon garlic powder

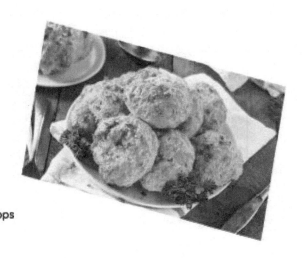

Instructions:
1. In a measuring cup, mix the heavy cream, vinegar, and enough water to make 1/2 cup. Let stand while you prepare the remaining ingredients.
   a. You may omit heavy cream, vinegar, and water and use 6 ounces of buttermilk instead.
2. Preheat the oven to 475°F / 246°C and line a baking sheet with parchment.
3. Sift the flours, baking powder, garlic powder, baking soda, and sugar together. Using your fingers, crush the salt as you add it to the flour.
4. Stir in the cheese.
5. Melt the butter.
6. When the oven is ready, add the liquids and butter to the dry ingredients. Mix until it just comes together. Mixture will become airy.
7. Quickly scoop 2 tablespoon (1oz) sized mounds onto the baking sheet.
8. Bake on the top rack for 14–20 minutes or tops and bottoms are golden brown. Rotate sheet halfway through baking time.
9. Melt the tablespoon of butter and mix with the salt and garlic powder. Brush the tops as soon as they come out of the oven.
   a. If desired, you could omit the cheese and garlic powder for plain biscuits.

Recipe tips:
- The number of biscuits you end up with, depends on how you measure out your flour.
- You can place regular granulated sugar into a grinder and pulse until it is a very fine consistency.
- Can sub with Bob's Red Mill® Gluten Free 1 to 1 baking mix for the flours.
- Sub nondairy cream, cheese, and butter.

Allergens:
Wheat/Gluten, Dairy. Cheese, if using.

Nutrition Information:
Calculated using the NB20 system which is linked to the USDA database. Not lab tested so nutrition is not lab accurate. Calculated using cake flour and caster sugar. Calculated for 12 biscuits.

Calories: 112, Fat: 8g, Sat. Fat: 5g, Trans Fat: 0g, Cholesterol: 23mg, Carbohydrates:8g, Fiber: 0g, Sugar: 0g, Sodium: 189mg, Protein: 2g, Calcium: 63mg, Phosphorus: 48mg, Potassium: 22mg

6

I'll Take the Next Category, Bob: Labels & Ingredients

Understanding Labels & Ingredients

Welcome to the only lesson in module six!
I am sure you are familiar with nutrition labels so this unit won't take long.

The first sheet is simply some tips and a quick mention of some things regarding the label.
As we know, phosphorus is not required on American labels. Potassium now is, and should be on there, but not everyone has caught up to it yet, which makes things more frustrating for us.

Another frustration is the crap they don't really have to tell you. The stuff they disguise with other words. I am talking about the wonderful world of hidden or not listed ingredients.

When you pick up any frozen or packaged meat product look for the bold boast or the fine prints about a "retained water solution" or something to that effect (Remember, we covered that in book one).
These solutions contain either/and/or potassium, phosphorus, and sodium. Frozen are often as high as 20% of these solutions. I can't even remember the last time I went near a frozen meat or meat product.

NOT great options.
We haven't bought them since starting this journey.
I had to ask my butcher at the meat counter to go pull their boxes and tell me the maker and what solutions and preservatives were used.
We found out who supplies the meat for our fresh meats counter, and they use a sodium and potassium preservative solution.

If you have a reputable butcher in your area, it may be a great time to get to know them. I can often get unseasoned, no salt added, no preservatives or solutions, meats there.
I can get unseasoned ground pork, unseasoned briskets, and I can also get a hold of those odd items like beef bones, marrow bones, and chicken feet to make amazing stock.
(Yeah, I have been making my own stock for years and I still get a little weirded out by the chicken feet).

When you are buying some of the "fresh" meats, make sure to buy the 4- or 5-ounce sized portions instead of the 8 or 12 ounces. It helps keep you closer to your serving amounts and no weighing or cutting later and it is easier to freeze the commonly used 1/2-pound portions.

Organic is always your safest and best option, but if it isn't available or is too pricey, find the product with the smallest "solution" amount listed on those labels.

For ground poultry, look for brands that utilize celery or rosemary as their preservative instead of potassium/phosphorus/sodium solutions. I believe Honeysuckle® and Jennie-O® have some.

Speaking of ground meat, in a recipe, unless it specifies a certain lean percentage, just use 80/20% or 85/15%. If a different percentage is required, it will state that.

Here's another situation…

Store made bakery items are usually high in sodium, they often use potassium and/or phosphates for preservatives and stabilizers.

Ask the department heads for nutritional information.

Sadly, I have yet to find a store's bakery department that can give me the nutritional info.

We learned to avoid that section, for the most part.

The only exception I have made is store bought mini croissants because, who wants to make them? not me! and those premade doughs that you can bake up are simply off the charts when it comes to sodium and preservatives. Good idea to bypass that section completely.

I am sure those mini croissants in the bakery are high in sodium and contain preservatives but, if you buy the mini size, be mindful of the (probable) increased minerals and adjust your remaining meals or snacks for the day, you should be fine.

You always have the option that if you cannot locate the information, avoid purchasing that product.

So, on your reference sheets I have listed a bazillion ingredients that you have probably seen more than once on the label.

These aren't things to necessarily watch out for, unless you have an allergy, sensitivity, or want to be very clean with what you put into your body.

Now you will see all the different uses for an ingredient and just how many there are!

Always look at the first three ingredients of a product. Those will help you gauge whether the product may be high in potassium or phosphorus. The ingredients listed on the label are always in order according to the amount used in making said product. The first ingredient is the largest or most abundant in that product.

I hope you can move some of these reference sheets to your phone cos (and here we go with the "in my day" story), when we started this journey, I was standing in the stores, with sheets and sheets of paper in my hand.

I hope people were thinking that I was a caterer or part of some TV show, cos that probably looked like a HUGE grocery list to them.

So much easier now!

READING LABELS

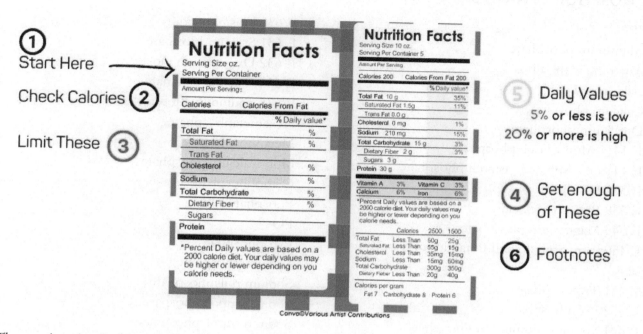

The serving size is always your starting place. Often the serving size will be ridiculous so you will have to calculate based on reality. Check calories if you need to watch them.

Note item 4. This is the section to look for Potassium, or sometimes Phosphorus to be listed as a percentage. Footnotes supply extra information that some people may need.

When looking at labels, Follow these guidelines:

- Avoid:
    - high sodium (200 milligrams or above) with potassium and/or phosphorus listed midway or high in the list of ingredients.
    - Potassium: over 251mg
    - Phosphorus: 300mg or more, or a percentage of 20% or more.
- Better:
    - lower sodium (between 140 and 200 milligrams) with potassium and/or phosphorus listed at the end of the list of ingredients, preferably after the "contains 2% or less" statement.
    - Potassium: 151-250mg
    - Phosphorus: 151-299mg, or a percentage of 15-19%.
- Best:
    - low sodium (under 140 milligrams), with no potassium or phosphorus added.
    - Potassium: under 150mg
    - Phosphorus: under 150mg, or a percentage of less than 15%.

There will be products, like soy sauce, that won't necessarily fit into these guidelines. The sodium is in the avoid category, but we know we will be using under the serving size amount.

NUTRIENT NAMES

PHOSPHORUS NAMES:

"P"
Aluminum phosphate
Anything with "Phos"
Baking powder
Calcium phosphate
Dicalcium phosphate
E 1410 Monostarch phosphate
E 1413 Phosphated distarch phosphate
E 322 Lecithins
E 338 Phosphoric acid
E 343 Magnesium phosphates
E 450 9a-c) Sodium and Potassium Phosphate salts
E 451 Triphosphates
E 452 Polyphosphates
E 541 Sodium Aluminium Phosphate
E 624 Monoammonium glutamate (MSG)
E 626 Guanylic acid
E 627 Sodium Guanylate
E 628 Dipotassium guanylate
E 629 Calcium guanylate

E 630 Inosinic acid
E 631 Sodium Inosinate
E 632 Dipotassium inosinate
E 633 Calcium inosinate
E 635 Sodium-5-Ribonucleotide
Hexametaphosphate
Metaphosphate
Monocalcium phosphate
Orthophosphate
Phosphate salt
PO4
Pyrophosphate
Sodium phosphate
Sodium polyphosphate
Sodium tripolyphospate
Sodium tripolyphosphate
Tetrasodium pyrophosphate.
Tribasic Magnesium Phosphate
Tricalcium phosphate
Trisodium phosphate

POTASSIUM NAMES:

Acesulfame potassium or Ace-potassium or Ace-K
Alkali potash or potassium
E 202 potassium sorbate
E 228 Potassium hydrogen sulphite
E 252 Potassium Nitrate
E 261 Potassium acetate
E 326 Potassium Lactate
E 332 Potassium Citrate
E 336 Potassium L-Tartrate (Cream of Tartar)
E 340 Potassium phosphates
E 450 (a-c) Sodium and Potassium Phosphate salts
E 451 Potassium malate
E 452 Triphosphates

E 470 Sodium, Potassium and Calcium Salts of Fatty Acids
E 501 Potassium carbonates
E 508 Potassium Chloride
E 950 Acesulfame K
Electrolyte
Kalium or "K"
Nitre/Nitrite
Potash
Potassium aspartate
Potassium bicarbone
Potassium carbonate (K2CO3)
Potassium gluconate
Potassium iodide
Potassium nitrate (KNO3)

Potassium oxide (K2O)

Potassium sulfate (K2SO4)

Potassium-magnesium sulfate (K2SO4-MgSO4)

Qali

Salt of petra

Salt peter

Saltpetre

Stone salt

SODIUM NAMES:

"Na"

Aluminum sodium sulphate (E 521)

Anything with "Sodium" or "Salt"

Ascorbyl palmitate (E304)

Baking soda/Sodium bicarb/ bicarbonate/bicarb of soda (E 500)

Brine

Calcium benzoate (E 213)

Calcium citrate (E 333)

Calcium disodium EDTA (E 385)

Calcium L-Ascorbate (E 302)

Calcium lactate (E 327)

Calcium propionate (E 282)

Calcium salts of fatty acids (E 470)

Calcium silicate (E 552)

Calcium stearoyl lactylate (E 482)

Cream of tartar (potassium L-Tartrate (E 336)

Cyclamic acid (and its Na & Ca salts) (E 952)

Dimethyl dicarbonate

Dioctyl sodium

Disodium phosphate

Gycine (and its sodium salt) (E 635)

Hydroxy benzoate salts (E 214-219)

Magnesium carbonate (E 504)

Magnesium silicate/Sodium aluminate (E 553)

Meat or Yeast extract

Monocalcium phosphate (calcium phophate monobasic)

Monosodium glutamate (MSG) (E 624)

Monosodium phosphate

N-Acetyl-L-methionine

Potassium benzoate (E 212)

Potassium chloride (E 508)

Potassium citrate (E 332)

Potassium lactate (E 326)

Potassium propionate (E 283)

Salt of lactic acid (E 270)

Sodim tetraborate; borax (E 285)

Sodium & potassium phoshphate salts (E 450 (a-c))

Sodium acetate (E 262

Sodium acid phosphate

Sodium adipate (E 356)

Sodium alginate (E 401)

Sodium aluminosilicate (sodium silicoaluminate, aluminium silicate) (E 554)

Sodium aluminum phosphate (E 541)

Sodium ascorbate

Sodium benzoate (E 211)

Sodium carboxymethylcellulose (cellulose gum) (E 467, 468)

Sodium chloride

Sodium citrate (E 331)

Sodium erythorbate (E 316)

Sodium ethyl p-hydroxybenzoate (E 215)

Sodium ferrycyanide (E 535)

Sodium flouride

Sodium gluconate (E 576)

Sodium Guanylate (E 627)

Sodium hexametaphosphate

Sodium hydrogen sulphite/bisulphite (E 222)

Sodium hydroxide (E 524)

Sodium inosinate (E 631)

Sodium L-Ascorbate (E 301)

Sodium L-Tartrate (E 335)

Sodium lactate (E 325)

Sodium lauryl sulfate

Sodium malates (E 350)

Sodium metabisulphite (E 223)

Sodium methyl p-hydroxybenzoate (E 219)

Sodium methyl sulfate

Sodium nitrite (E 250), nitrate (E 251)

Sodium orthophenyl phenol (E 232)

Sodium phosphate

Sodium phosphate (E 339)
Sodium polyacrylate-acrylamide resin
Sodium potassium tartrate (E 337)
Sodium propionate (E 281)
Sodium propyl p-hydroxybenzoate (E 217)
Sodium pyrophosphate
Sodium saccharin
Sodium silicoaluminate
Sodium sorbate (E 201)
Sodium stearate

Sodium stearoyl lactylate (E 481)
Sodium stearyl fumarate
Sodium sulf - ate, ide, or ites (E 221), (E 514)
Sodium sulfo-acetate deriviatives (mono- & diglycerides)
Sodium tribasic phosphate
Sodium-5-Ribonucleotide (E 634)
Sorbic acid
Starch sodium octenyl succinate (E 1450)
Stock cube/powder

PROTEIN NAMES:

Albumin
Algae
Alpha-lactalbumin
Amino acids
Artichoke
Asparagus
Bean & nut flours
Beans
Beta-lactoglobulin
Broccoli

Brussel sprouts
Calcium caseinate
Casein
Caseinates
Protein Names:
Albumin
Algae
Alpha-lactalbumin
Amino acids
Artichoke

Asparagus
Bean & nut flours
Beans
Beta-lactoglobulin
Broccoli
Brussel sprouts
Calcium caseinate
Casein
Caseinates

LABEL:

Salt/Sodium Free: less than 5mg per serv

Very Low: 35mg or less per serv

Low/Lower: 140mg or less per serv

Reduced: at least 25% less sodium than regular item

Light or Lightly Salted: at least 50% less than the regular item

No Salt Added or Unsalted: none added during processing (doesn't mean it is absolutely salt free unless stated)

INGREDIENTS

For those with allergens or who simply want to know what the ingredients are.
This is not a complete list as there are too many to mention.
For CKD, take note of all the various potassium, phosphorus, & sodium items there are!
View the video here: https://youtu.be/dmV4lXaphzc

- **Acidity Regulators**: control Ph levels. Sodium salts, Sorbic acid, Acetic acid, Benzoic acid, Propionic acid.

- **Acidulants**: impart a tartness. Acetic acid, Ascorbic acid, Citric acid, Fumaric acid, Lactic acid, Malic acid, Phosphoric acid, Tartaric acid.

- **Algae/Seaweed**: Agar, Carrageenan, Alginate, Beta carotene, brown, red, bue-green, or green algae, Spirulina, Chlorella, Nori, Kelp, Dulse, Eukaryotic phyla of rhodophyta, Chlorophyta, Phaeophyta, Bacillariophyta, Dinoflagellates, Prokaryotic phylum of cyanobacteria, Microlage, Algal hydrocolloids, Alginic acid and salts, Ammonium alginate, Calcium, Potassium, and Sodium alginate, Alginic acid, Algin, Propylene glycol alginate.

- **Anticaking Agent**: Tricalcium phosphate, Powdered cellulose, Magnesium stearate, Sodium bicarbonate, Sodium, Potassium, or Calcium ferrocyanide, Bone or Calcium phosphate, Sodium silicate, Silicon dioxide, Calcium silicate, Magnesium trisilicate, Talcum powder, Sodium or Calcium aluminosilicate, Potassium aluminium silicate, Bentonite, Stearic acid, Polydimethylsiloxane.

- **Bulking Agents**: starches: Dextrin, Maltodextrin, Glucose syrups, Corn syrups, Dextrose, Fructose syrup, Sugar alcohols: Maltitol, Erythritol, Sorbitol, Mannitol, Hydrogenated starch hydrolysate. Modified starches: Dextrin, Acid or Alkaline treated starch, Bleached or Oxidized starch, Enzyme treated starch, Monostarch phosphate, Distarch phosphate, Acetylated distarch phosphate, Starch acetate, Hydroxyprpyl starch, Starch sodium octenyl succinate, Resistant starch, Synthetic starch.

- **Cheese**: see milk.

- **Citrus**: Bioflavonoids, Citrus peel, Ehyl 4, 4-dichlorobenzilate, Lime, Lemon, grapefruit, n-octanoic acid, Caprylic acid, Oleic acid, Palmitic acid, Pentaerythritol ester of maleic anhydride modified wood rosin, Petigrain lemon, mandarin, or tangerine, Citrus aurantium, Propylene glycol alginate.

- **Corn and Derived From**: Ascorbic acid, Cornstarch, Caramel color, Calcium citrate, Cellulose, Citrate, Magnesium citrate, Potassium citrate, Sodium citrate, Citric acid, Dextrin, Maltodextrin, Dextrose (can be in meat, lidocaine, and novocaine), Honey baked items, Ethanol, Ferrous gluconate, Artificial or natural Flavorings, Golden syrup, corn syrup, Honey, Hydrolyzed vegetable protein (HVP), Iodized salt or other salts, Lactic acid, Magnesium stearate, Malic acid, Malt, Malt flavoring, Maltitol (Maltisorb or Maltisweet), Mannitol, Modified food starch, Monosodium glutamate (MSG), Polydextrose, Polysorbates, Powdered sugar, Saccharin, Sodium Erythorbate, Sodium starch glycolate, Sorbitan, Sorbitan monostearate, Yeast, Sorbitol, Starch, Sucralose, Sweet'N low, Tocopherol, Vanilla extract, Vitamins, Xanthan gum, Sylitol, Maize, Zein.

- **Dough Conditioners**: Ascorbic acid, Monoglycerides, Diglycerides, Ammonium chloride, Enzymes, Amylase, Protese, Lipoxygenase, Carbamide, Urea, Malted barley, DATEM, Potassium bromate, Calcium salts, Calcium iodate, L-cystine, Glycerol monostearate, Azodicarbonaminde, Sodium stearoyl lactylate, Sucrose palmitate, Sucrose ester, Polyoxyethylene sorbitan monostearate, Polysorbate, Soybean lecithin, Ammonium sulfate, Ammonium phosphate, Phosphoric acid, Cysteine, Bisulfite, Fumaric acid, Sodium bisulfite, Sodium metabisulfite.

- **Eggs**: Albumin, Albumen, Apovitellin, Globulin, Lecithin, Ovalbumin, Ovovitellin, Lysozyme, Surimi, Mayonnaise, Egg white protein, Egg white powder, Egg substitute, Dried egg solids, Egg yolk, Egg wash, Eggnog, Fat substitutes, Livetin, Meringue, Meringue powder, Ovoglobulin, Ovomucoid, Ovomucin, Ovotransferrin, Ovovitelia, Ovovitellin, Powdered eggs, Sili Albuminate, Simplesse, Trailblazer, Vitellin, Artificial flavor, Natural flavor, Pasta.

- **Fish & Seafood**: Fish protein concentrate, Fish protein isolate, Isinglass, Fish liver oil, Roe, Marine oil, Ocenaol, Oleths, Oleyl arachidate, Oleyl imidazoline, Pristane, Ambergris, Sqalene, Shark liver oil, Sponge, Luna, Sea, Turtle oil, Vitamin A, Vitamin D3, Fish gelatin, Worcestershire sauce, Anchovy, Caviar, Omega-3.

- **Food Coloring**: Quinoline yellow, Carmoisine, Ponceau 4R, Patent blue V, Green S, Brilliant blue FCF, Indigotine/Indigo, Fast green FCF, Erythrosin, Allura Red AC, Tartrazine, Sunset Yellow FCF, FD&C blue 1 and 2, FD&C Green 3, FD&C Red 2, 3, 4, 32 and 40, FD&C yellow 1, 2, 3, 4, 5 and 6, Citrus red 2, Orange B, FD&C orange 2, FD&C Violet 1, Azo, Xanthene, Pyrazolone, Indigoid, Triarylmethane, Carotenoids, Chlorophyllin, Anthocyanins, Betanin, Annato, Caramel coloring, Carmine, Cochineal, Achiote, Elderberry, Lycopene, Paprika, Turmeric, Curcumin. Color retainers: Sodium bisulfite, Ascorbic acid.

- **Flavorings**: Manzanate, Diacetyl, Acetylpropionyl, Acetoin, Isoamyl acetate, Benzaldehyde, Cinnamaldehyde, Ethyl propionate, Methyl anthranilate, Limonene, Ethyl decadienoate, Allyl hexanoate, Ethyl maltol, 2,4-Dithiapentane, Ethylvanillin, Methyl salicylate, Glutamic acid, Gycine salts, Guanylic acid, Inosinic acid, Ribonucleotide salts.

- **Glazing Agents:** Stearic acid, Beeswax, Candelilla wax, Carnuba wax, Shellac, Microcrystalline was, Crystalline wax, Lanolin, Oxidized polyethylene wax, Esters of colophonium, Paraffin.

- **Gluten:** see wheat

- **Humectants:** used to keep moisture. Propylene glycol, Hexylene glycol, Butylene glycol, Aloe vera, Alpha hydroxy acids, Lactic acid, Egg yolk or white, Glyceryl triacetate, Honey, Lithium chloride, Molasses, Polymeric polyols, Polydextrose, Quillaia, Sodium hexametaphosphate, Sugar alcohols, Glycerol, Sorbitol, Xylitol, Maltitol, Urea, Castor oil.

- **Milk:** Casein, Caseinates, Lactalbumin, Lactoferrin, Lactulose rennet casein, Whey, Yogurt, Cream, Ghee, Cheese, Whey protein, Whey isolate, Milk protein, Buttermilk, Cultured milk, Buttermilk solids, Condensed milk, Dried milk or solids, Evaporated milk, Milk powder, Goat's milk, Lactaid milk, Lactic acid, Malted milk, Milk derivative, Milk protein, Milk paste, Sheep's milk, Sweet cream, Sweetened condensed, Dairy protein, Butter flavor, Butter extract, Butter fat, Butter solids, Ammonium caseinate, Calcium caseinat, Hydrolyzed casein, Iron caseinate, Magnesium caseinate, Potassium caseinate, Sodium caseinate, Zinc caseinate, Natural or artificial cheese flavor, natural or artificial cheese food, Imitation cheese, Casein, Curds, Custard, Dairy product solids, Galactose, Half & half, Hydrolysates, Sherbet, Lactalbumin, Lactate solids, Lactitol monohydrate, Lactoglobulin, Lactose, Anhydrous Milk fat, Pudding, Quark, Recaldent, Rennet, Simplesse, Sour cream solids, Imitation sour cream Yogurt powder, Acid whey, Cured whey, Delactosed whey, Dimineralized whey, Hydrolyzed whey, Whey solids, Natural flavorings, Flavoring, Caramel flavoring, High protein flour.

- **Mushrooms:** Myco, Mycelium, Mycelia, Mushroom, Spore, Fungi, Fungus, Dried mushroom powder, Mycoprotein.

- **Peanuts:** Arachis, Arachis oil, Nut pieces, Nut meal, Peanut butter, Peanut flour, Beer nuts, Boiled peanuts, Peanut oil, Crushed nuts/peanuts, Earth nuts, Goober peas, Ground nuts/peanuts, Hydrolyzed peanut protein, Hypogaeic acid, Mandelonas, Monkey nuts, Nu nuts, Nutmeat or pieces, Peanut paste, Peanut syrup, Peanut sauce, Spanish or Virginia peanuts, Artificial flavoring, Chili, Crumb topping, Egg rolls, Enchilada sauce, Fried foods, Graham cracker crust, Hydrolyzed plant protein, Hydrolyzed vegetable protein, Marzipan, Mole, Natural flavoring, Nougat. Ethnic foods: African, Asian, Chinese, Indian, Indonesian, Thai, Vietnamese, Mexican. Possible reaction to: Lupin bean, Lupinus albus, Soybean.

- **Preservatives:** antimicrobials: Sorbic acid, Sodium sorbate, Benzoic acid, Benzoates, Parabens, Sulfur dioxide, Sulfites, Nitrites, Nitrates, Lactic acid, Propionic acid, Propionates, Phosphoric acid, Isothiazolinones (MIT, CMIT, BIT), Formaldehyde releasers (DMDM hydantoin). Fat preservatives: Ascorbic acid, Sodium ascorbate, Butylated hydroxytoluene, Butylated hydroxyanisole, Gallic acid, Sodium gallate, Sulfur dioxide, Sulfites, Tocopherols, Mono/polyphenol oxidase, Citric acid.

- **Salt**: anything with the words sodium or salt. Sodium nitrate, citrate, benzoate, Monosodium glutamate (MSG), Baking powder or soda, Seasoning, Brine, Broth, Stock, Percent solution, Enhanced, Natural flavoring, Disodium, Meat/Yeast extract, Bouillon, stock, or broth cubes and powders.

- **Shellfish**: Abalone, Calamari, Caracoles, Clams, Cockle, Crab, Crawfish, Crayfish, Crawdad, Crevette, Escargot, Langouste, Langoustine, Lobster, Mollusks, Mussels, Octopus, Oysters, Prawns, Scallops, Scampo, Shrimp, Snails, Squid, Squid ink, Krill, Bouillabaisse, Cuttlefish, Cuttlefish ink, Fish stock, Seafood seasoning, Glucosamine, Surimi, Ecrevisse, Scampi, Coral, Tomalley, Cherrystone, Littleneck, Pismo, Quahog, Barnacle. Geoduck, Limpet, Lapas, Opihi, Periwinkle, Sea cucumber, Sea urchin, Whelk, Turban shell, Fish sauce, Oyster sauce.

- **Soy**: Edamame, Hydrolyzed soy protein, Miso, Natto, Shoyu, Soya, Soybean, Soy protein, Soy isolate, Soy sauce, Tamari, Tempeh, Textured vegetable protein (TVP), Tofu.

- **Stabilizers**: also see preservatives. Alginate, Agar, Carrageen, Cellulose, Gelatin, Guar gum, Gum Arabic, Locust bean bum, Pectin, Starch, Xanthan gum, Tara gum.

- **Sugars**: Agave and nectar, Barbados, Barley malt and syrup, Beet, Molasses, Brown, Buttered syrup, Cane juice, crystals, solids, sugars, or syrups, Caramel, Carob syrup, Castor, Coconut and/or Palm, Confectioner's Powdered, Baker's, Superfine, Corn sweetener, syrup, or solids, Crystalline fructose, Date, Demerara, Dextran, Dextrin, Dextrose, Diastatic malt, Diastase, Oat syrup, Ethyl maltol, Evaporated cane juice crystals, juice, syrup, or sugar cane, Florida crystals, Free flowing brown, Fructose and crystals, Fruit juice concentrate and crystals, Galactose, Glazing, Glucose solids and syrups, Golden sugar and syrup, Granulated, Grape, Gum syrup, High fructose corn syrup, Honey, Icing , Invert sugar and syrup, King's syrup, Lactose, Malt sugar and syrups, Maltodextrin, Maltol, Maltose, Mannose, Maple syrup, Muscavado, Nectar, Pancake syrup, Panocha, Raw, Refiner's syrup, Rice syrup, Saccharose, Simple syrup, Sorbitol, Sorghum syrup, Sucanat, Sucrose, Sweet sorghum, Syrup, Treacle, Turbinado, White, Xylose, Yellow.

- **Thickeners/Emulsifiers**: Mono- & diglycerides, Sodium phosphates, Diacetyl tartaric acid esters of mono– and diglycerides (DATEM), Cellulose, Mucilage, Soy lecithin, Polysaccharides, Starch, Gums, Pectin, Arrowroot, Cornstarch, Katakuri, Potato, Sago, Tapioca, Polymers, Guar, Locust bean gum, Carob bean, Agar, Aginin, Carrageenan, Xanthan, Collegen, Gelatin, Casein, Food additives, Stabilizers, Natural gums, Alginic acid, Sodium alginate, Potassium alginate, Ammonium alginate, Calcium alginate, Brown algae, Glucomannan, Konjac, Aiyu, Ice jelly,

Potassium chloride, Natural ingredients, Dextrin, Hydrochloric acid, Sodium or Potassium hydroxide, Hydrogen peroxide, Sodium hypochlorite, Maltodextrin, Cyclodextrin, Phosphoric acid, Sodium or potassium phosphate, Sodium triphosphate, Distarch phosphate, Sodium triphosphate, Acetic anhydride, Hydroxypropylated starch, Ether, Propylene oxide, Hydroxyethyl starch, Ethylene oxide, Succinate, Cationic starch, Monochloraecetic acid, Phoshphated distarch phosphate, Acetylated distarch adipate, Hydroxypropyl distarch phosphate.

- **Tree Nuts**: Almond, Brazil, Caponata, Cashew, Chestnut, Filbert, Gianduja, Hazelnut, Hickory, Macadamia, Marzipan, Almond paste, Nougat, Nut butter, Nut meal, Nut flour, Nut oil, Nut paste, Nut pieces, Pecan, Pesto, Pine nuts, Pistachio, Praline, Walnut.
- **Wheat**: Bran, Breadcrumbs, Bulgur, Couscous, Cracker meal, Durum, Farina, Flour, Gluten, Kamut, Matzo, Matzoh, Seitan, Semolina, Spelt., Wheat protein, Protein isolate.

TASK

Welcome to your module six task.

So here we are, coming in from our pleasant walk, feeling refreshed, and sitting down to dive into our task.

Yep, it's task time.

This week, please grab the Nutrient Calculations sheet from the last unit and do some calculations on some condiments you have in your home.

- Calculate out for 2 teaspoons, 5 teaspoons, and 7 teaspoons, try calculating the percentages from some of the labels too.

This won't take too long, and you should feel like a pro afterwards.

Then continue and calculate out a few more items you have been curious about.

- Lastly, if you really want to be ambitious, grab a recipe you enjoy. Perhaps a pre-CKD recipe, or maybe one you found online or in a magazine. Calculate the entire recipe and see where you can make changes or go ahead and make those changes and plan to use the recipe in an upcoming week.

This is the process you want to use when adapting or even creating a recipe.

- If potassium is too high, start reducing or swapping the high potassium ingredients.
- If phosphorus is too high, start reducing or swapping the high phosphorus ingredients.
- Again, the same for high sodium, protein, carbs, etc.
- Make these adjustments, and if needed, swap until it falls in line.
- If you made a lot of reductions, look at options for adding bulk back in.

Then, because you probably had to reduce sodium, as we always do, head on over to the spices sheet and see what you can add in to bump up flavor or add a bit more of each spice. Choose the spices based on the largest ingredient amounts in the dish, we want them to work with the main ingredients, like chicken, or beans.

When we reduce sodium, we will often use a combination of at least three different spices. Heck, I have a recipe that has 7!

The more you do this, the easier it gets and the better you become. One day you will look at a recipe and instantly have an idea of whether it will be too high in potassium, or phosphorus, protein, carbs, sodium, etc. AND, you will have an idea how to adjust it too!

Believe me, if you keep at this, you will get there. I promise.

Now, I am not making the recipe calculation a required task this week as you have covered a lot thus far. And you probably still need to finish your subs list too, which we will be using in the next module.

But I am going to highly encourage you, and well, downright beg, that you please do this.

It will only help you to solidify the info in your mind and make you even better at this.

This will also help you to understand how to adapt or even create recipes.

If you just don't have the time, that is ok. Come back to this later when you are ready to adapt or create recipes.

When you have finished, let's head over to our first Action week where you will be doing daily tasks.

Get your subs list ready!
Ok, maybe take one more relaxing walk before diving in.

Happy Calculating!

7

Let's Try Meal Planning for $200

THE CORE METHOD

Are you ready to get this ball rolling?

First up, we are going to walk you through how to breakdown and solidify your personal daily base guideline meal and snack numbers.

This is the key to helping you pick recipes and menu plan. It also is key in helping you to adapt any recipe, so it fits within your numbers.

This keeps you on track, and your kidneys happy.

Don't worry, we are going to show you how to adjust those numbers when you are having a BBQ, at a family gathering, meeting friends for brunch, or a big holiday arrives with all the amazing foods.

YES! You are going to see how you can indulge during the holiday and adjust your daily meal and snack numbers so you can stay reasonably close to your daily limits.

Once you have your numbers, you will be picking recipes that you will adapt and then prepare.

Make sure you grab book one, cos we will be using those databases!

Grab your personal list of foods that you created cos we're using that too.

Then we will close out this first part of the core method with a breakdown of how to tally up your weekly menu numbers, so you know that everything falls into line, you know your allotment amount for snacks each day, and…… no more daily tracking!

I have to tell ya, this is the exciting part! This is where the magic happens that starts you on the road to building an arsenal of recipes that are tailored to your (and your family's) needs.

When this arsenal is built, you can keep adding to it but more importantly, your kidney diet becomes crazy, in-freaking-sanely easy. (That's a technical word, by the way. Ha!)

Pick your recipes for the day, do a quick tally, know your nutrient availability for snacks, make your grocery list, and shop.

Done.

Crazy. Freaking. Easy.

Set to your needs, fits your restrictions, no stress, no worries, no searching.
Just enjoying a tasty kidney diet.

Hey, that's been your goal all along, right?

Here's your chance to make it happen!

Happy Goal Reaching!

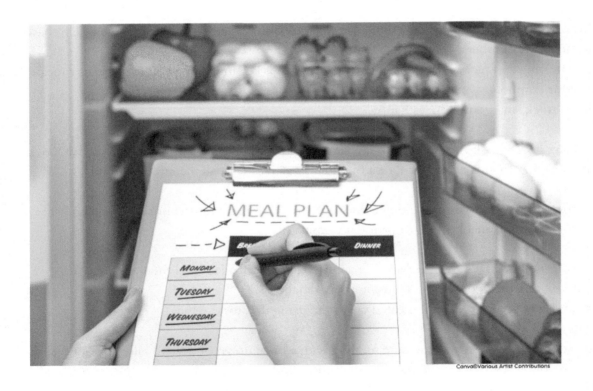

YOUR PERSONAL BASE GUIDELINE MEAL & SNACK NUMBERS

Okay, we are walking through this but don't worry, I am giving you a visual sheet as well. Read through this first to get a basic understanding, then look over the sheet.

- Start by listing out the daily restrictions you have.
    - For example, my hubby's restrictions look like this: potassium is 1900, phosphorus is 900, and Sodium is 1900.
    - Everyone's numbers can be different. Make sure you have talked with your dietician. If you are in stage 2, 3, 4, or 5 and they say you don't have restrictions, I suggest getting a second opinion.
- Now list what you eat each day, starting with the biggest meal.
    - For example: ours is dinner, then lunch, then breakfast, then snacks. If desserts are a regular part of a meal, say at dinner, then include them with dinner.
- Now, we want to create some guideline numbers that you will be looking for when finding recipes.
    - You want to assign percentage numbers to the larger meals. You can use any numbers you want to use as long as it all adds up to 100%.
        - For example: Our biggest meal is dinner. We want a larger number because higher amounts of those nutrients will be consumed. We assign 35%.
        - Next is lunch. Because we use the leftover portions from dinner the night before, we know that we must have 35% for lunch.
            - If you have a smaller lunch, like a simple salad or sandwich, you can make your lunch number smaller.
        - Then we looked at breakfast. Breakfast is very small, if eaten at all. So, we only assigned 15%.
        - We are snacky people who like to graze so we want to assign enough to cover those. So, we assigned 15%.

We have our numbers and now we need to translate that into guideline nutritional numbers.

Potassium and sodium are 1900 mg per day, and we want 35% available for dinner and lunch so, multiply. 1900 x 35% (0.35) = 665. (Remember that sheet in the Math section with helpful conversions? Peek at that if you need to know the decimal form)

When looking at the nutrition in a recipe, we do not want the potassium and sodium amounts to exceed 665 mg. Under is fine, but don't go over.

Phosphorus is 900.
900 x 0.35 = 315. We will look for recipes that also do not exceed 315 mg of phosphorus.
Continue to calculate each nutrient you need to track by the percentage.

When finished, you should have your list.

Again, make sure to include all nutrients that you must restrict.
You should end up with a little chart that you can keep handy each time you are looking for recipes.

Let's find your numbers!

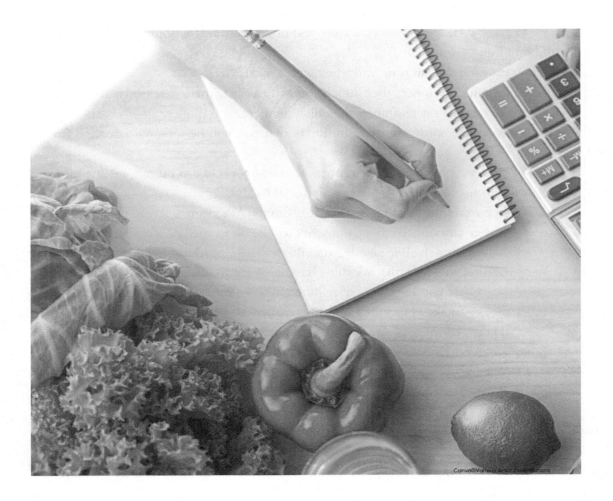

VISUAL FOR FINDING YOUR NUMBERS

- **First**:
  - List your daily restrictions. Include any other nutrients you must track.
    - For example:
      - Potassium 1900mg
      - Phosphorus 900mg
      - Sodium 1900mg
- **Second**:
  - List the meals you eat each day. We include snacks so we make sure to have room for them. Desserts will be counted in with the meals they are eaten with. Basically, consider the dessert as part of your meal.
    - For example: Breakfast, Lunch, Dinner, Snacks
- **Third**:
  - Assign a percentage to each meal. Give more to the larger meals of your day.
    - For example:
      - Dinner 35%
      - Lunch 35%
      - Breakfast 15%
      - Snacks 15%
- **Fourth**:
  - Find your base guideline numbers.
    - For example: your potassium limit is 1900, dinner is set at 35%
      - 1900 x 35% (0.35) = 665 milligrams of potassium max.
  - Continue to calculate your restricted nutrients and percentages until you have your chart of your maximum nutrient amounts per meal.
-
  - **EXAMPLE**:

	Dinner (35%)	Lunch (35%)	Breakfast (10%)	Snacks (15%)
Potassium	665	665	285	285
Phosphorus	315	315	135	135
Sodium	665	665	285	285

This process is going to become second nature after you have gotten the hang of it.

Keep going! Move on to the next step.

MENU PLANNING

Okay, now that you have done steps 1-4 to find your numbers, here is where we start menu planning and adapting.

Let's continue with the next steps (5 through 7)

- **Fifth:**
  - o ***Add this step once you begin your CKD cooking journey. For now, jump to step six so you can learn the process first.**

    (This is the portion that helps you use up those leftovers)
    - ▪ Take inventory of leftovers you need to use up. See if you can use them in a recipe you have chosen.
      - ▪ If you have half a red pepper left, use that in your eggs one morning. If you have 1/2 pound of chicken left, use that instead of ground beef (if it works in the recipe). Then you don't need to buy ground beef.
      - ▪ If you have decided to double a meal place a sticky note on it to remind you when creating your shopping list.
      - ▪ If you use a leftover meal as your lunch, use a place holder sheet to remember it, with the nutritional info per serving for your restricted nutrients.
      - ▪ If you will take the suggestion and have your non-CKD person do an Italian sausage and leftover stew, put Italian sausage on your white board now.

- **Sixth**:
  - o Find CKD recipes that contain nutritional information.
    - ▪ Here are some suggested sites. You can also search "kidney disease recipes" to find even more sites.

American Kidney Fund's Kidney Kitchen https://kitchen.kidneyfund.org/

Davita https://www.davita.com/diet-nutrition/recipes

National Kidney Foundation https://www.kidney.org/recipes-search

NW Kidney Centers https://www.nwkidney.org/living-with-kidney-disease/recipes/

Fresenius https://www.freseniuskidneycare.com/eating-well/recipes

Diabetes Food Hub https://www.diabetesfoodhub.org/all-recipes

- If you have side dishes or accompaniments, those will reduce the amount of the main dish.
  - o If I choose a chili recipe and want biscuits on the side, I must make sure that the chili and biscuit combined will add up to my guideline amount of 665 potassium, 665 sodium, and 315 phosphorus.
- Now, gather one week's worth of recipes and print them out. Select enough for one week plus 1 or 2 more that have slightly lower nutritional values in case you need to make changes.

- o If you are having a side dish or dessert with a meal, place them together as they are one meal.
- Create a placeholder sheet for odd items that you do not have a recipe for. For example, a piece of toast with jam.
  - o Look up the nutrient amounts in the USDA database (or pull the info from the product) for those nutrients you must track and note them on the placeholder sheet. Also put a sticky note onto the recipe itself to remind yourself to add in that nutrition into the total of the recipe nutrition.
  - o Make sure it falls in line with your allotted numbers per meal.

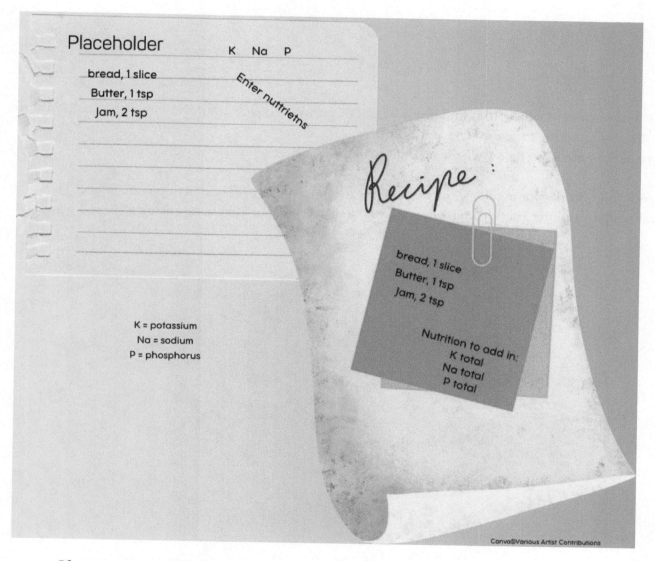

- If you are using dinner as lunch the next day, create a placeholder sheet with the name and restricted nutritional info on it, per serving.

- **Seventh**:
  - o Place your chosen recipes and placeholder sheets into daily piles.
  - o You should now have each day in their own respective piles, and have all placeholder

sheets within, and desserts grouped with the meals they will be eaten with or placed in the snacks pile.

- o   When you begin listing the items on your tally sheet, you will have the info you need for each day and the placeholder sheets will remind you of that item, and the necessary nutritional info, per serving, listed and ready use.

If you would like to view the video, go here: https://youtu.be/Qv_EZatUPKw

Okay, now that we have that under our belt, let's address those situations where you need to shift your base guideline meal and snack numbers.

This is the process to follow when you want to indulge or have a holiday or gathering.

Once you rework your numbers, run through the menu planning to assure all things are in line. Then you will head over to the Tallying unit where we will double check our intake and ensure all is well.

REWORKING YOUR NUMBERS

Perhaps you are going to a family brunch and that brunch will now be your biggest meal of the day. Maybe you found a recipe you must try but the nutrients are above your basic guidelines.

- Then, let's adjust!
    - Locate the nutritional info for your restricted nutrients on the recipe.
    - Calculate the new percentages for the day.
        - For example: your base guideline potassium is 665 per serving.
            - You will be indulging in an enchilada dish that has 760 potassium per serving.
            - Find the percentage: 760 (amount in recipe) divided by your daily restriction 1900.
                - 760 / 1900 = 0.4 (move decimal over **two places to the right**) 40%.
            - The new percentage for dinner on this happy enchilada day is now 40%.
    - Reassign percentages to remaining meals.
        - For example
            - Our dinner we know is 40%.
            - Because our lunch is the leftovers from dinner the night before, we know it must stay at 40%.
            - Breakfast we will reduce to 10% and we are keeping snacks at 10% cos we love to snack!
- Knowing these numbers, calculate all restricted nutrients according to the new percentages to create your numbers for that day.

EXAMPLE

	Dinner (40%)	Lunch (40%)	Breakfast (10%)	Snacks (10%)
Potassium	760	760	190	190
Phosphorus	360	315	90	90
Sodium	760	760	190	190

You now have your new base guideline numbers for that day, so you can enjoy that slightly higher potassium meal!

Okay, now we need to take a step to remind ourselves of this change, now and in the future.

- On your enchilada recipe, place a sticky note with your new percentage that you must stick to on that day.
  - Next time you pull it out to make it, those new guideline numbers are there to remind you.
- Make sure to include this on your placeholder sheet too, Ya know, if you are having some of those enchiladas for lunch the next day.
  - This will remind you that you need to stick to those percentages on the day you have them for lunch.

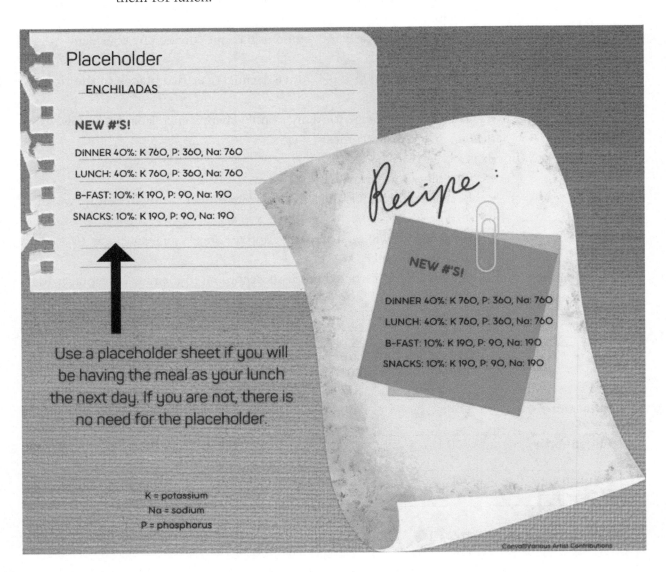

Placeholder

ENCHILADAS

NEW #'S!

DINNER 40%: K 760, P: 360, Na: 760

LUNCH: 40%: K 760, P: 360, Na: 760

B-FAST: 10%: K 190, P: 90, Na: 190

SNACKS: 10%: K 190, P: 90, Na: 190

Use a placeholder sheet if you will be having the meal as your lunch the next day. If you are not, there is no need for the placeholder.

K = potassium
Na = sodium
P = phosphorus

Recipe :

NEW #'S!

DINNER 40%: K 760, P: 360, Na: 760

LUNCH: 40%: K 760, P: 360, Na: 760

B-FAST: 10%: K 190, P: 90, Na: 190

SNACKS: 10%: K 190, P: 90, Na: 190

Canva/Various Artist Contributions

ADAPTING RECIPES

Are you still with me? You are doing great!

Here is what we need to do with our recipes next.

We need to take those chosen recipes for each day and adapt them for any allergens or dislikes or maybe swap them for alternatives like vegan meats.

Here's a quick run through...

Start with day 1 recipes and note any ingredients that you need to swap.

Grab your reference sheets and your subs list; this is where you are thankful you did it!

Go through each recipe and note your substitution on the recipe along with the amount you will be subbing.

If you will not be using something from your subs list, use your veggie sheets to find alternatives.

Here, I could look at the vegetable swaps sheet and see that a good swap for butternut squash is pumpkin, acorn squash, sweet potatoes, yams, or carrots.

Then head on over to the vegetable sheets and find the charts. Look at each of those suggestions and decide which one you want to use.

Winter squash (butternut) is in the High Potassium column under starchy vegetables.

You can replace it with another item from that list or one from the medium or low potassium lists.

If you are watching carbs, head over to the non-starchy lists and choose something from there.

You don't need to look up info if you are swapping from the same potassium amount column unless you want to be super accurate. If you sub in sweet potatoes for that butternut squash, you already know it is in the high potassium category and numbers will be similar.

If you are making a swap for something from the lower potassium columns, you can look it up in the USDA and decide if you can add more. Or you can simply leave it, knowing the potassium will be a bit lower.

If you do look it up in the USDA, you can recalculate the nutritional information of your restricted nutrients based on any changes you made.

This will simply let you know if you have some extra potassium or other nutrients that you now have a little extra of. You could then add that to your snack allotment and have some slightly higher potassium snacks, or you can use a little more of an ingredient in your recipe.

This is the process that will help you to allow for more snacking, or, more importantly, add bulk to those small-portioned meals.

So, for example, the recipe says 1/2 cup of butternut squash, you want to sub a non-starchy veggie like green beans.

1/2 cup of butternut has 247 mg of potassium.

1/2 cup of no salt added canned green beans has 65 mg.

247 (potassium from squash) – 65 (potassium from green beans you will use) = 182 milligram reduction in potassium.

You can now decide if you want to use the 182 mg of potassium on snacks or if you want to raise the amount of green beans you are using.

Keep going!

Here, we are going to raise the beans to 1 cup.

Note the change like this...

- Cross out butternut and next to it write: No Salt Added Canned Green beans, **1 cup**, Potassium: **130**, Phosphorus: 58, Sodium: 3.

- Now subtract the 1 cup green beans substitute's potassium amount from the squash potassium amount,

    - 247—**130** = 117.

- Note the difference in parenthesis (-117 potassium) on your recipe. Do this for all restricted nutrients.

- Then you can look at the potassium listed in the nutritional info on the recipe and minus the 117 from the total. That is the new potassium amount in the recipe.

    o Cross off the old potassium amount and note the new number above it.

You have the info available from now on and can type it up nice and pretty too.

You now have the new potassium amount listed and this helps with choosing recipes later.

Take this step by step as you go through. By the end, you should feel pretty comfortable with this process.

So, go through all your recipes and make those swaps. Use the heck out of your reference materials, that is exactly what they are there for! To make this as easy as freaking possible.

Okay, let's run through this one more time so it really makes sense to you.

Walk through these step-by-step and get comfortable with the process before moving on.

- **First:** Locate any items on the recipe that you need to swap.

- **Second**: Use any reference sheets needed to find an acceptable substitute.

  - Note that substitute on the recipe, along with the amount you will be subbing with.

- **Third**: If your chosen ingredient substitute falls within the same column as the original ingredient (the one you want to replace), you can just note the change (cross off okra and write your alternate). The nutrition will be similar enough.

  - OPTIONS

    - If your chosen alternative is lower in potassium, you can look up the item in the USDA and decide if you want to use a bit more of it, or simply leave it; knowing the potassium in the dish will be a bit lower.

    - If you choose an ingredient that is higher in potassium, you will need to look it up in the USDA and figure out how much to reduce the amount by. Often reducing it by half helps.

      - If you've chosen to reduce the amount you are using because it is higher in potassium, remember, you may need to raise another ingredient to replace the amount you are removing, or add something in.

        - Let's say you cut your higher potassium ingredient in half, from 1/2 cup to 1/4 cup. There is now 1/4 cup of food missing from the recipe. This may result in smaller portions and hungry tummies. (Keep going, we will cover this too!)

- **Fourth**: If you are simply making an ingredient swap. **If you did look it up** in the USDA, you can recalculate the nutritional info of your restricted ingredients and write it on your recipe.

    - Do the calculation (1/2 cup okra is 108 potassium, canned green beans, 1/2 cup, is 63, difference is 45).

      - Decide if you will put that 45 potassium into snacks or if you want to leave it as is or make adjustments.

    - Here, we are going to raise the beans to 1 cup. Note the change like this...

      - Cross out okra and next to it write canned green beans, 1 cup, Potassium: 147, Phosphorus: 30, Sodium: 3 (include all nutrients you must track).

      - Now subtract the okra potassium amount from the 1 cup green beans' potassium amount (147—108 = 39).

        - *We subtracted the okra from the beans because we increased the beans. Had we not increased the beans, we would subtract the beans from the okra, resulting in a reduction in potassium (-45).*

- Note the difference in parenthesis (39 potassium) on your recipe. Do this for all restricted nutrients. then add up all the changes, negative or positive.

- Then look at the potassium listed in the nutritional info section on the recipe and add the 39 from that total. This is the new potassium amount in the recipe.

- Cross off the old potassium amount and note the new number above it. You have the info available from now on, and you can type it up too.

- You now have the new potassium amount listed and this helps when meal planning later.

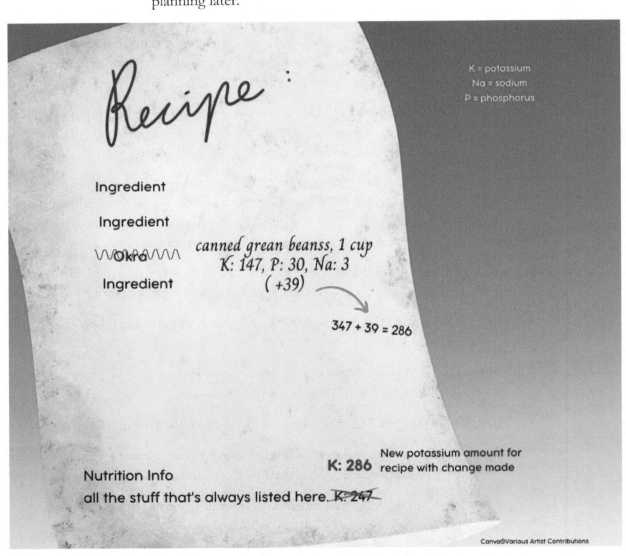

How did you do?

This is an extremely important piece for ease and success of the kidney diet.

Use this!

I promise you, there will come a point where you won't need to refer to this and will simply look at a recipe and know instantly what change to make and about how much.

You WILL get there!

If you would like to see a visual walkthrough you can go here: https://youtu.be/BIyyeiwB_Mk

Okay, let's move on and discuss that situation of adding in bulk.

Keeping Bulk in Your Meal

- If you made your adaptations and had to reduce something, you can now look for something to replace it.

    o For example, if you reduced your beef, look at the grains sheet, we know grains contain less protein and phosphorus than meat. Choose an item from the low phosphorus and low potassium columns. At the top of that sheet, it states 3 1/2 ounces, so you could add in grains for that 1/4 lb. of protein you removed.

Let's go into this a bit more...

- Let's say you have a recipe that you are dropping the meat from 1 pound down to 1/2 pound. Now, you need to replace those 8 ounces of food you've removed.

    o First, make the note on your recipe for the meat change, subtracting from the protein, phosphorus, potassium, and sodium amounts listed in the recipe (include all nutrients you must track).

    o Now, find an 8-ounce replacement that is lower in protein, phosphorus, sodium, etc.

        ▪ Let's use Shiitake mushrooms. They are a great "meaty" sub.

            ▪ Find the nutrition for 8 ounces. Make the notes for the nutrition on the recipe, then adjust the total nutritional numbers. Your recipe is now set.

Let's address this situation that can arise.

If you make the swap and now find your potassium is too high, we need another adjustment.

        ▪ You can cut the mushrooms to 4 oz instead, and add 4 oz of grains, or pasta.

            ▪ You will note the nutrition for 4 oz of mushrooms, and for 4 oz of grains or pasta on your recipe.

            ▪ Then do your final tally of the total nutrition so you now have the recipe set.

Another example: If you are reducing vegetables, see the vegetables sheet and find the column it is in.

- For example, you want to reduce potassium, so you remove carrots from the recipe entirely.

    o On the starchy vegetables sheet, it shows the potassium range for carrots to be 151-250mg.

        ▪ Now you can choose a lower potassium veggie, or you can look at something different, like pasta.

- Pasta contains around 60-70mg of potassium per 1 cup cooked, you could add in 1 cup of pasta and have now reduced some of the potassium in your dish but replaced it with another ingredient to keep the bulk in the recipe.

This may seem confusing at first, or like a lot of work but I promise you, this becomes super easy once you are familiar with the process. Just keep at it!

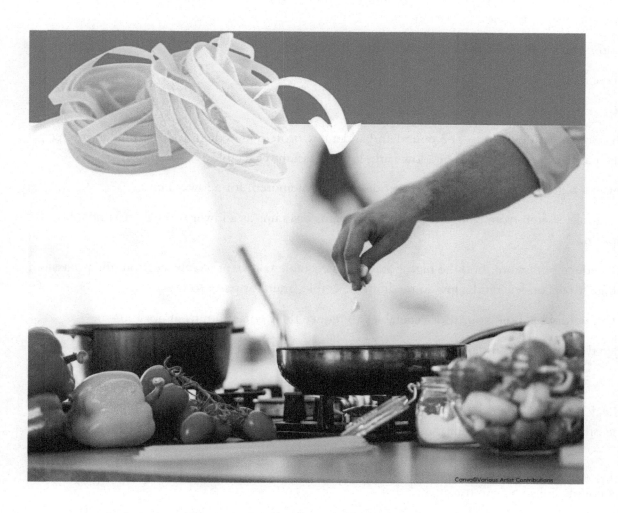

STAGES & LABS

LABS

When you get your labs back, if they show an issue with something being too low or too high, you can adjust.

Depending on your stage and restrictions, adjust your recipes to fall in line with what you need.

Increase

- Raise your protein or phosphorus by adding more meat, dairy or beans. Add more vegetables into the dish to increase potassium.

- Add more snacks, side dishes, or desserts.

- Have a bigger portion.

Decrease

- Reduce protein by 1/4 to 1/2 pound and add a low protein ingredient to keep bulk in the recipe like pasta, rice, or couscous or a low carb, low potassium vegetable.

- Swap a high potassium, phosphorus, sodium, or protein item for a lower item.

- Example, switch from using ground beef to beans or grains as a lower protein and phosphorus option.

- To reduce potassium, find the high potassium vegetable you want to replace, note the potassium range it falls under. Find a low to medium vegetable, grain, or pasta to use.

- Dialyze (double boil) your root vegetables to reduce their potassium by almost 50%.

- Use the tips from our dairy unit. More fat = less phosphorus. Or use a non-diary product.

Always check nutrition when subbing an alternative product like plant-based meat, dairy, low carb, or gluten free products. The ingredients and nutrition vary immensely, so note all nutritional changes.

Here are a couple links you can use also:

A USDA Nutrition Value Guide PDF:
www.ars.usda.gov/is/np/NutritiveValueofFoods/NutritiveValueofFoods.pdf

A Canadian Value Guide PDF: https://www.canada.ca/content/dam/hc-sc/migration/hc-sc/fn-an/alt_formats/pdf/nutrition/fiche-nutri-data/nvscf-vnqau-eng.pdf

STAGES

Protein

- If protein is too high, reduce proteins in your meals like Meat, Beans, Whole grains, and/or Dairy. Sub with a lower protein items like pasta, refined grains, or another lower protein item.

- If protein is low, increase them.

- Add a few tablespoons of chopped nuts to your dish. Use whole grains or lower phosphorus beans. Add higher protein snacks.

Potassium

- If potassium is too high, reduce potassium in your meals. Meat, Beans, Nuts, Grains, Vegetables, Fruits. Swap for a lower potassium item.

- If potassium is too low, increase them or add snacks.

- Swap for a high potassium item.

Phosphorus

- If phosphorus is too high, reduce phosphorus in your meals. Meat, high phosphorus beans and whole grains, nuts, dairy.

- If phosphorus is too low, increase them. Add high phosphorus snacks. Use more cheese!

Sodium

- If Sodium is too high, reduce the amount you use and increase your use of acidic ingredients.

- Add lemon juice at the end of the meal, serve with a citrus wedge to squeeze over top, use one of the suggested salt replacers (Mr. Dash, Benson's, True Lime/Lemon, etc.).

- Use other items to replace high sodium ingredients. Example, use low sodium products but use a combination of products to mimic the taste. Example: using a combination of soy sauce, Worcestershire sauce, coconut aminos, and vegan fish sauce to lower the amount of sodium.

- If sodium is too low, increase sodium in recipes by 1/8 to 1/4 teaspoon. Recheck labs. Adjust again.

HELPFUL QUICK ADAPTING GUIDE

The amounts suggested are based on the following guidelines:

Potassium: 600mg or less per serving, per meal.

Phosphorus: 300mg or less per serving, per meal.

Sodium: 400mg or less per serving, per meal.

Protein: can range from 2g to 40g per serving, per meal.

If you are allowed more or less than the guideline amounts listed, you can **make adjustments** by increasing or decreasing amounts. As always, consult your doctor or dietician.

****These are suggested guidelines.**

They are <u>not</u> guaranteed to fit your exact needs.

Some things you can use more or less; it will depend on your specific recipe and needs.

In my unscrambling and creating, I found these patterns to be rather consistent.

Still, these do not always fall true.

This is simply a quick guide/guideline to use in a pinch.

Use these guidelines as you see fit.

The recipe adapting and creating you have learned will yield more true results. **

4-Serving Recipes

- **VEGETABLES**

    o   If using 3 different vegetables, use 1/2 cup of each.

    o   More than 3 vegetables, reduce to 1/4 cup each.

- **FRUITS**

    o   If served fresh as a side, limit to 1/4 cup per person with the meal.

    o   If served fresh as a snack, 1/2 cup.

    o   If you are incorporating fruit into a dish, limit it to 2 tablespoons of chopped dried fruits such as raisins, cranberries, or apricots. Limit to 1/2 cup when baking.

    o   Limit to 1/2 cup fresh in a dish or 1 cup when baking.

- **MEATS**

    o   Use 1/2 to 3/4 pounds, depending on other proteins or high phosphorus ingredients in the dish.

    o   If you are using a low amount of other proteins or phosphorus ingredients, use 3/4 pound, otherwise stick to 1/2 pound.

    o   Use lower amounts if combining with beans or a significant amount of dairy. For example, if you are making chili, use 1/2 pound of meat with 1/2 cup of beans, if you are also using dairy.

    o   Use 1/2 pound of meat with 3/4 cup of beans if you are using very little dairy or none.

- **DAIRY**

    o   Use a maximum of 1/4 cup of dairy such as sour cream, crème fraiche, cream cheese, and plain yogurts.

    o   Use a maximum of 1/2 ounce of cheese per person in a 4-serving dish. Look for the lowest sodium you can find.

    o   Use strong flavored cheeses.

- **EGGS**

    o   Stick to 2 eggs per meal.

- **NUTS & SEEDS**

    o   Nuts should be limited to 2 tablespoons. Chop for the best texture and distribution.

    o   Seeds should be limited to 1 tablespoon.

- **BEANS**

  o Use 1/2 cup beans with 3/4 pound of meat.

  o Use 3/4 cup of beans with 1/2 pound of meat.

  o If not using meat, you may be able to add up to 2 cups, depending on the other proteins and high phosphorus ingredients in your dish.

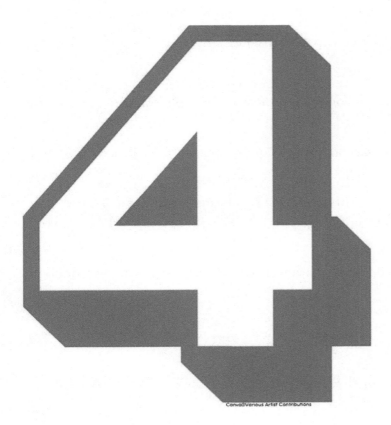

Canva@Various Artist Contributions

6-Serving Recipes

- **VEGETABLES**
  - If using 3 different vegetables: use 3/4 cup each.
  - More than 3 vegetables, reduce to 1/2 cup each.

- **FRUITS**
  - If served fresh as a side, limit to 1/4 cup per person with the meal.
  - If served fresh as a snack, 1/2 cup.
  - If you are incorporating fruit into a dish, limit it to 2 tablespoons of chopped dried fruits such as raisins, cranberries, or apricots. Limit to 1/2 cup when baking.
  - Limit to 1/2 cup fresh in a dish. Limit to 1 cup when baking.

- **MEATS**
  - Use 1 to 1 1/4 pounds, depending on other proteins or high phosphorus ingredients in the dish.
  - If you are using a low amount of other proteins or phosphorus ingredients, use 1 1/4 pound. Otherwise stick to 1 pound.
  - Use lower amounts if combining with beans or a significant amount of dairy. For example, if you are making chili, use 1 pound meat with 1 cup of beans, if you are also using dairy.
  - Use 1 pound of meat and 1 1/2 cups of beans if you are using very little dairy or none.

- **DAIRY**
  - Use a maximum of 1/2 cup of dairy such as sour cream, crème fraiche, cream cheese, and plain yogurts.
  - Use a maximum of 1 ounce of cheese per person, look for the lowest sodium you can find. Use strong flavored cheeses.

- **EGGS**
  - Stick to 2 eggs per meal.

- **NUTS & SEEDS—**
  - Nuts should be limited to 3 tablespoons. Chop for the best texture and distribution.
  - Seeds should be limited to 1 tablespoon.

- **BEANS**

- o Use 1 cup beans with 1 pound of meat if also using dairy.

- o Use 1 1/2 cups of beans with 1 pound of meat if using very little dairy or none.

- o If not using meat, you may be able to add up to 3 cups, depending on the other proteins and high phosphorus ingredients in your dish.

Canva@Various Artist Contributions

Other Food Categories

- **GRAINS**

  - Use up to 2 cups cooked, if the dish is largely grain-based.

  - Use 1 to 1 1/2 cups cooked if the dish is about equal amounts of grains and other ingredients.

  - Use 1 cup cooked, if being used as a component, and not a main ingredient.

  - Use up to 1/2 cup cooked, if using as a filler for more bulk.

- **PASTA**

  - Should be kept at 2 ounces, dry, per person.

- **GROUND AND DRIED SPICES**

  - Contain potassium and phosphorus.

  - Most often used amount is 1 teaspoon, but to compensate for low sodium, can use up to 2 tsp.

  - Some seasonings, like chili seasoning or taco seasoning may use up to 2 tablespoons, just double check the ingredient list for potassium additives. If so, limit to 1 - 1 1/2 tbsp and increase other ingredients within the mix, like cumin.

  - Easy tip: simply bump up the seasonings in the recipe when you decrease the salt. Takes the guesswork out of what to use!

- **FRESH HERBS**

  - Contain potassium but it is not as concentrated as dried, so you can use more of it than dried or ground.

  - If it has a woody stem, add to the dish early.

  - If it does not have a woody stem, use it at the very end or as a garnish.

- **SALT**

  - 1 teaspoon of kosher (coarse grain) salt contains 1,760mg of sodium.

  - 1 teaspoon of table salt contains 2,330.

    - Save yourself 570mg of sodium by switching to kosher. Anytime you need to, you can crush or grind it, or put it into liquids to dissolve first.

  - Try to keep to 1/8 to 1/4 teaspoon of kosher salt, depending on other high sodium ingredients. Very rarely will I use over 1/8 tsp, unless I know for certain that it fits in the recipe restrictions.

- **FATS**
  - Utilize healthy fats most often but don't sacrifice flavor!
  - The all-around best option is Olive oil.
  - However, feel free to use oils to impart flavor like sesame or peanut.
  - If using high heat, use equal parts butter and oil. This prevents the butter solids from burning.
  - Use refined oils for high heat and cooking.
  - Use unrefined, virgin, and extra virgin for low heat or for dressings.

- **VEGAN / VEGETARIAN**
  - Can sometimes contain more protein, sodium, phosphorus, and potassium, depending on what the product is made of. Other times, it can be less and work perfectly in your dish.
  - Base the amount you will use off the sodium and potassium per serving.
    - Check the ingredients list for "phos" ingredients. If it is high in the list, put it back. If it is listed under the "contains 2% or less" section, it should be fine. Allergens are common.

- **NON-DAIRY PRODUCTS**
  - Base your amounts on the potassium and sodium listed per serving.
    - Check the ingredients list for "phos" ingredients. If it is high in the list, put it back. If it is listed under the "contains 2% or less" section, it should be fine. Allergens are common.

- **GLUTEN FREE PRODUCTS**
  - Make sure the label says certified gluten free.
  - Base your amounts on the potassium and sodium listed per serving.
    - Check the ingredients list for "phos" ingredients. If it is high in the list, put it back. If it is listed under the "contains 2% or less" section, it should be fine. Allergens are common.

- **LOW CARB PRODUCTS**
  - Can contain high amounts of dairy, meats, cheese, and potassium ingredients.
  - Always use a lower potassium vegetable when swapping it for rice, pasta, beans, or grains.

o Check the ingredients list for "phos" ingredients. If it is high in the list, put it back. If it is listed under the "contains 2% or less" section, it should be fine. Allergens are common.

Now, enjoy the Bonus Crepes Recipe as a reward for kicking A$$!

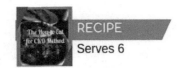

RECIPE
Serves 6

Easy Crepes

Ingredients:

3 ounces flour or gluten free flour (about 1/2 cup plus 1 tablespoon)
1/8 teaspoon coarse grain salt
1/2 cups water
3 large eggs
1/2 cup heavy cream or nondairy
2 tablespoons unsalted butter, melted and cooled or nondairy

Instructions:

1. Sift flour in a bowl. Dissolve the salt in the water. Melt butter and set aside.
2. Whisk the salted water, eggs, and cream. Add the flour and mix until combined.
3. Slowly whisk in the melted butter. Batter should be thin and may have small bits.
4. Heat an 8 to 10-inch pan over med-low heat until it is hot (water droplets will sizzle when thrown in the pan).
5. Remove pan from the heat, brush lightly with butter and pour 1/4 cup of batter into the pan. Slowly swirl the pan to spread the batter thin.
6. Put the pan back on heat and cook about 2 minutes, until lightly browned and top looks set. Crepe should be easy to flip. (cooking time will vary, depending on the size of your pan and thickness of your crepes).
7. Flip over and cook the second side, 45 seconds to 1 minute. There should be some browning. Slide onto a plate.
8. Do not oil the pan again unless crepes begin to stick. Repeat with remaining batter.
9. Fill with desired ingredients, roll and serve.

Recipe tips:

- May omit salt to reduce sodium to 44mg per crepe.
- Mix whipped strawberry cream cheese with whipped cream for a sweet filling. Top it with some fresh mint too!
- Fill with a mixture of sautéed vegetables and, if desired, diced low sodium bacon or sausage for savory.
- Spread 1 tablespoon of lower sodium peanut butter per crepe as a protein-based snack.
- Use gluten free flour and let batter rest 10 minutes before using.

Allergens:

Eggs, Dairy, Wheat/Gluten.

Nutrition Information:

Calculated using the NB2O system which is linked to the USDA database. Not lab tested so nutrition is not lab accurate. Calculated using first listed ingredients. Does not include fillings. Per crepe:

Calories: 186, Fat: 13g, Sat. Fat: 8g, Trans Fat: 0g, Cholesterol: 129mg, Carbohydrates:12g, Fiber: 0g, Sugar: 1g, Sodium: 124mg, Protein: 5g, Calcium: 32mg, Phosphorus: 78mg, Potassium: 65mg

TALLYING YOUR NUMBERS

First:

- Print or create a tally sheet for each day of the week.

- Grab a pencil and write day 1 or Monday in the top left box.

- In the boxes under the nutrients, list your daily restriction amounts. If you do not have a restriction for something, leave it blank. You don't need to worry about tracking it.

  - If you are unsure of your restrictions, head on back to module 1 for general nutritional guidelines and follow those until you have your personal ones.

Second:

- Start with your day 1 and choose the biggest meal of the day, for us, that is dinner. That is the one that will probably take up more of your nutrients than any of the others.

- Write dinner and list the meal and each of the nutrient amounts you must track.

- Write any side dishes or accompaniments and their nutrient amounts also.

- Now total up the amounts for that entire meal, include desserts too. Then subtract it from your daily total.

- Write the total you have remaining for each nutrient.

Third:

- Move to the next biggest meal of the day, this one is usually lunch for us. This one will probably take up the next biggest portion of your nutrients. As mentioned, to cut down on cooking and calculating, we have dinner from the day before.

- Now, write lunch and list the meal and each of the nutrients you must track. Write any side dishes or accompaniments also.

- Now total up the amounts for that meal. Then subtract it from your remaining daily total that you had leftovers from the first entry.

- Write the total you have remaining for each nutrient.

Fourth:

- Now choose your smallest meal of the day, this one is breakfast for us. This will take up a small amount of the nutrients for the day.

- Write breakfast and list the meal and each of the nutrient amounts you must track.

- Write any side dishes or accompaniments also.

- Now total up the amounts for that meal. Then subtract it from your remaining daily total from the previous meal.

- Write the total you have remaining for each nutrient.

Fifth:

- List and track your snacks.

- Now total up the amounts for those snacks. Then subtract it from your remaining daily total from the previous meal.

- Write the total you have remaining for each nutrient.

- Now tally to see how well you did for the day. Repeat for the remaining days.

- If your numbers did not fall in line, let's look at options.

IF YOUR NUMBERS ARE UNDER OR OVER:

OVER

- Look at the extra recipes you picked out and see if there is one that has a lower amount of the nutrients you need to reduce and switch. Then do a quick recalculation.

- If need, switch it with a different day's recipe.

- Look at your accompaniments, side dishes, and desserts. What can you trim down? Half a piece of cake? 1/4 cup of green beans instead of 1/2 cup? Simplify your side dish by having green beans with hollandaise instead of green bean casserole? Only 1 biscuit?

- Simplify a meal. No big egg bake, just a scrambled egg and English muffin.

- If needed, drop that lunch that was yesterday's dinner. Freeze it for emergency days and find a different recipe or have a simple lunch.

UNDER

- You can switch to a higher nutrient recipe or add extra snacks into that day.

- You could eat a bigger portion or increase some of your ingredients in the dish.

  - For example, if your potassium for the day was low, add in another 1/4 to 1/2 cup veggies to help get your potassium numbers up some.

- The goal is to remain as close as possible to your restrictions. It is fine to be within 50 milligrams over or under.

- The point of all this is to get you to reduce the amounts you used to consume. Being exact on the numbers is not mandatory. Being close, IS.

- Some recipes just cannot be lowered, like the enchiladas I had mentioned previously. For those, recalculate your meal and snack numbers for a higher nutrient day.

Have a look at the example sheet to help you out.

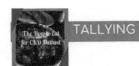

Tally Sheet

Monday	Potassium	Phosphorus	Sodium	Protein	Carbs	Fluids
Limit Per Day	1900 mg	900 mg	1900 mg	60 g	none	none
Dinner						
Chili	393	166	122	10		
Side of fruit	54	9	1	1		
Vanilla Souffle	127	104	101	10		
TOTAL:	**574**	**279**	**224**	**21**		
	1900-574 = 1326 mg left					
Lunch						
Bread roll	54	46	32	4		
Soup	349	212	158	17		
TOTAL:	**403**	**258**	**190**	**21**		
	1326-403 = 923 mg left					
Breakfast						
Egg bake	248	178	110	12		
Coffee w/ 2 T heavy cream	29	18	0	0		
TOTAL:	**277**	**196**	**110**	**12**		
	923-277 = 646 mg left					
Snack						
Veggies & dip	177	15	5	2		
Pasta Salad	102	43	153	3		
TOTAL:	279	58	158	5		
	646-279 = 367 mg left					
Totals for the day:	**1533**	**791**	**682**	**59**		
	Potassium	Phosphorus	Sodium	Protein	Carbs	Fluids

CKD Culinary Consulting

GROCERIES & PRODUCTS FOR CKD

You made it!

You now have one week's worth of recipes that are adapted, sorted, and tallied.

You are now ready to make your grocery list.

You can (Hopefully) take a picture of the grocery list template that I have created for you, where I have placed a very large list of items that would be good choices. It's amazingly helpful to have that on-hand while in the store.

When we first started shopping for CKD, I really struggled to know which foods or products were better choices than others.

Or when reading ingredient lists, which ingredients were better options or which to avoid.

I have taken all the low phosphorus or low potassium items and have listed all of them out on the back of this sheet. This way if you're standing in the grocery store and are unsure of what the better option might be, you can refer to it.

Keep in mind that although some of these might be lower in potassium, they might be a little higher in phosphorus, or if they're higher in phosphorus they might be a little lower in potassium but overall, these items should be your best options.

Because alternative products like low carb, gluten free, alternative meats, and dairies are really another world of their own, you really need to read the ingredients lists because they are all so greatly different.

You know, you read it all in book one!

So as not to neglect those categories, I instead listed some items that we use and that you can look for, either at your grocers or online.

Always, always keep in mind your allergens, even if I have listed products or brands or recommended them, please read the label and ingredients to make sure they do not contain anything that will harm you.

Here's another tip!

Manufacturers will often change the recipe of their products. I don't know if maybe they found a cheaper way to make that product, so they switch things around, but it happens.

One day, that product you regularly buy suddenly has too much sodium or they added potassium preservatives or phosphates to it.

So even though I commonly buy something, I will always double check the label every time just to make sure it's satisfactory before buying it. This also helps when I grab the product, start reading and see the sodium is off the charts. I turn it over and see that I grabbed the one next to it by mistake.

To make shopping faster and easier and so you don't have to go back and find something, organize your grocery list into sections. Clump all dairy together, all meat together, etc.

If you know your store well, you can even put the groupings in order on your sheet to match the layout of the store.

Ya know, I have no idea why I never did this for myself in the beginning but here we are and I'm glad I can offer this to you.

When you are ready, let's head on over to the next module.

Man, you are cruising through this. Way to go!

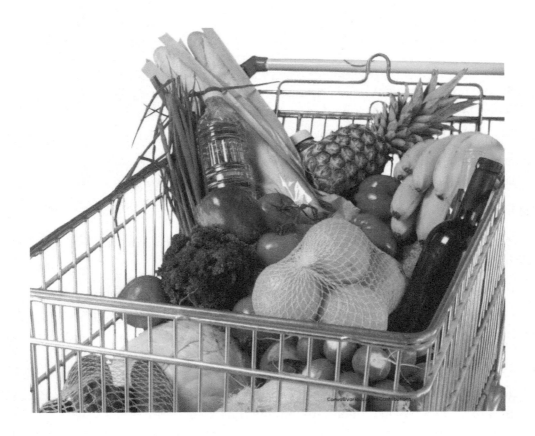

Fruits: Acerola, raw, frozen
Apples, canned, frozen, raw
Apple juice (not potassium added)
Applesauce, canned
Apricots, canned
Apricot nectar, canned
Blackberries, canned, frozen
Blackberry juice, canned
Blueberries, canned, frozen, raw
Boysenberries, canned, frozen
Cantaloupe, raw, frozen
Carambola (starfruit)
Cherries, maraschino, canned
Cherries, sour red, canned, frozen
Cherries, sweet, canned
Cranberries, dried, raw, frozen
Cranberry sauce, jellied or whole
Cranberry juice
Figs, canned, raw
Fruit cocktail, canned
Gooseberries, canned
Grape juice
Grapefruit juice
Grapefruit, raw, canned, frozen
Guava nectar, canned
Jackfruit, canned
Kiwano, raw, frozen
Lemons, juice and zest
Limes, juice and zest
Loganberries, frozen, raw
Lychee, canned, raw, frozen
Mango nectar
Mangosteen (a berry, not mango), canned
Olives, canned/jarred
Papaya, canned
Papaya nectar, canned
Peach nectar, canned
Peaches, canned, frozen
Pears, Asian, raw, frozen
Pears, Bosc
Pears, Red & Green Anjou
Pears, canned, raw, frozen
Pear nectar
Pineapple, frozen, canned, raw
Plums, canned
Rambutan, canned
Raspberries, canned, frozen
Rhubarb, frozen
Guanabana (soursop, graviola, guayabano) nectar
Star fruit (carambola)
Strawberries, canned, frozen
Tamarind nectar, canned
Tangerines / mandarins, canned
Watermelon, raw, frozen

Veggies:
Bamboo shoots, canned
Bean sprouts (mung), canned, raw
Beans, green (snap, string, wax), canned, raw, or frozen
Cabbage, napa, raw

Capers, jarred
Cauliflower, raw, frozen
Chayote, raw
Collard greens, raw, canned
Cucumber, raw
Eggplant (aubergine), raw or pickled
Garlic & Ginger, raw
Grape leaves, canned
Iceberg lettuce, raw
Jicama (yambean), raw
Kale, frozen, raw
Leeks, raw
Lettuce, Iceberg
Mushrooms, canned
Mushrooms, Shiitake, raw
Mushrooms, Straw, canned
Mushrooms, Jew's ear (pepeao), raw
Okra, raw
Olives, green or black
Onions, frozen, raw
Peppers, green chili, canned
Peppers, hot, red or green, pickled, canned
Peppers, bell, frozen, canned
Pickles, sweet or sour, low sodium
Radish sprouts, raw
Seaweed, Irish moss, raw
Seaweed, kelp, raw
Seaweed, wakame, raw
Turnip greens, canned, frozen
Turnips, raw or frozen
Water chestnuts, canned
Zucchini, yellow (summer squash), canned
Beets, pickled, canned
Corn, sweet yellow or white, creamed or canned
Hominy, white, canned
Hominy, yellow, canned
Peas, green, canned, frozen
Squash, winter (butternut), frozen

Nuts & Seeds:
Quinoa
Edamame (soy beans)
Wild rice
Chia seeds, raw
Macadamia
Hickory nuts, raw
Walnuts, raw
Walnuts, dry roasted
Chestnuts, boiled, steamed, raw
Pili nuts
Pecans
Egg Noodles
Semolina, Wheat, Rice, Whole grain, Corn & Rice based pasta

Cheese:
Blue (soft)
Brie (soft)
Burrata
Camembert (soft)

Cottage cheese
Cream cheese
Farmer
Feta
Goat cheese
Goat's milk (chevre)
Gorgonzola
Mascarpone
Mozzarella
Neufchatel
Paneer
Panela
Processed American
Quark
Queso blanco
Queso fresco
Ricotta
Sheep's milk, fresh

Grains:
amaranth
barley, pearled
buckwheat groats
bulgur, cornbran
cornmeal, couscous
farro, hominy
khorasan wheat
millet, oat bran
quinoa, rice, all
semolina, spelt
teff, wheat, sprouted
wild rice

Legumes:
tofu, fried
peanuts, boiled
tofu, extra firm, cooked
tofu, soft, cooked or raw
tofu, firm, cooked or raw
peanuts, dry roasted or raw
chickpeas, canned
adzuki, canned
kidney, red, canned
pinto, canned
lupini, boiled
blackeyed peas, canned
Refined **oils** for cooking
Unrefined or virgin for dressings and low temp cooking
Arrowroot

Flours: Corn flour, meal, starch
All-purpose, bread, cake, pastry flour
Light Rye flour
Millet flour
Quinoa flour
Refined Sorghum flour
White Rice flour
Semolina flour
Tapioca flour
Fava flour
Cassava flour

Other Suggestions:
Mrs. Dash seasonings and packets, marinades, etc.
True Lime, True Lemon seasoning blends
Benson's table tasty
Orrington Farms low sodium beef and chicken broth powders
Chocolates with the first three ingredients being unsweetened chocolate, sugar, and cocoa butter.

Vegan/Vegetarian options:
Check sodium!
Quorn meatless grounds
JUST egg replacement
Beyond meat, some products ok to use
Lightlife tempeh bacon and hot dogs
Silk non dairy products
Follow your heart veganaise and other products
Amy's Kitchen canned beans

Gluten free: Enjoy Life, Mi-DEL, Kinnikinnick, Glutino, Goodie Girl, Schar, Lucy's, Bob's Red Mill 1 to 1 gluten free flour mix with xanthan

Avoid: high sodium (200 milligrams or above) with potassium and/or phosphorus listed midway or high in the list of ingredients.
Potassium: over 251mg, Phosphorus: over 300mg, or a percentage of 20% or more.

Better: lower sodium (between 140 and 200 milligrams) with potassium and/or phosphorus listed at the end of the list of ingredients, preferably after the "contains 2% or less" statement.
Potassium: 151-250mg, Phosphorus: 151-300mg, or a percentage of 15-19%.

Best: low sodium (under 140 milligrams), with no potassium or phosphorus added. products like soy sauce are exceptions.
Potassium: under 150mg, Phosphorus: under 150mg, or a percentage of less than 15%.

8

Organizing & Shopping for $250, Please

Here we go!!
Now that you've worked through the process that has you on the path to CKD eating freedom, let's keep it going with the second part of the core method.

This section is a little more supplemental but equally important.

Let's get you organized.
No, not like moving furniture or clearing your browser history.
Organized like, making it easier to use up any leftover ingredients, which can be super common with CKD eating.

To make a recipe work, oftentimes, we max out at 1 cup of beans, and since most standard cans contain 1 1/2 cups, we now must figure out what to do with that extra 1/2 cup.
We don't really want to throw it away, that's money in the trash.

We are also going to help you organize your system, so you always know, at any second of the day, what you need to pick up from the grocery store.
No more digging around and wondering if you still have that can of diced green chilis.

And we are going to help you work out how you can prepare for those days when cooking just isn't going to happen.

So, when you are ready, let's get you going.

Happy Organizing!

ORGANIZING

Welcome to the organizing section where I am going to give you a few more tips. I am just going to start throwing them towards you. Hopefully some of them stick!

- Whiteboard, dry erase markers, magnetic clips, calculator.
  - o As mentioned, keeping a magnetic whiteboard, markers, and clips on your fridge will help you keep organized by noting items you run out of.
  - o Clips help hold your recipes. One for the recipes to be cooked, the other holds the ones that have been cooked.
  - o The whiteboard really helps when you want to go into your fridge and take inventory of any leftovers or any leftover ingredients that you want to use up. You can make notes on your whiteboard of what these are and then choose recipes based off those for the coming week to use them up.
- I highly suggest having a calculator handy in the kitchen. I keep a magnetic shelf on the side of my fridge that holds my calculator, paper, pens, my freezer tape, and permanent markers, and maybe some manuals from kitchen gadgets.

- You may or may not have leftover ingredients, however it frequently happens. Because of restrictions, oftentimes you'll see recipes that call for one cup of beans or a half a cup of beans or maybe a quarter cup of celery or a half pound of ground beef. All these leftover items need to be used up.
  - o You could use vegetable scraps or leftover vegetables to make stock, which you can also freeze, by the way.
  - o When you make your own stock, it really brings a depth, roundness, and fullness that you can't get from store-bought. It really is worth the time to make. They're fantastic for things like French onion soup. You can also make stock in an InstaPot® now too! Ok. enough about stocks.
  - o Use veggies in quick breakfasts or lunches by making omelets, small salads, or make stock and freeze it.
  - o Another option is to buy some Italian sausage and have the non-CKD person make a soup or stew with all the remaining leftovers. We have come up with some fantastic stuff doing that. So, plan to buy some Italian sausage too!
  - o Create your own dish using them up on the weekend. Do some quick calculations of each leftover ingredient or simply have a "cheat day" and enjoy the Italian leftovers soup with your non-CKD person.
  - o Freeze them or use fruits and veggies in compost or toss out for wildlife to eat.

That step #5 I had you jump over and said we would be returning to it. Here's where you will see how to incorporate it.

- Organize your shopping list by sections. Group them together by department. If possible, list those groups according to the layout of your store.

- Coordinate with sales when planning meals to save money.
- You can actually freeze buttermilk, cream, half-and-half, egg yolks and egg whites.
  - So, if you purchase something, say buttermilk, it often happens that you only need 1/2 to 1 cup, and you still have at least a half a container left. Portion that out and freeze it.
- Do you have a carton of eggs that you aren't going through quickly? You can separate the whites and the yolks and freeze them also.

- <u>Keep a running list of those items you freeze so you know what you have.</u>
  - We have a second, larger whiteboard next to our chest freezer with all the contents listed. When we use something or add to it, we note it on the board.
  - This will help when making grocery lists too. What's been in there a while that we need to use? What do we need to buy? Ground beef? got it! Don't need to buy more. Just need to remember to take it out in time.
    - I then placed a sticky note on that recipe to remind us to take the beef out. Each day I glance forward to see if there are any upcoming reminders like that on my recipes.

- Now, remember to note on your grocery list, one or two subs for produce that will be acceptable. Sometimes stores are out of stock. Be prepared.

- Sometimes, ok, super often, when I need parsnips, carrots, or turnips, they are only offered in a bag. Great. I now have six turnips and only need one.
  - Either choose a sub or make a note on your white board when you get home that turnips need to be in next week's recipes. You could use those turnips as subs for other veggies in next week's recipes to use them up.
  - Call up friends and family and see if they could use some and swap them for something else, maybe you only need 1 large carrot next week, swap them for one.

- Speaking of family and friends, if you are newly diagnosed, here are some options:
  - Flipping your kitchen and pantry over to all new products can be an undertaking. So, ask family and friends to help.
  - Let them know you have three cans of black beans and ask them to pick up some low sodium or no salt added cans the next time they shop, and swap with them.

As it happened, when my hubby got diagnosed, we had just shopped the day before. We had bags of stuff we couldn't use. Bags!
I told our kids and family to pick up certain no salt or low sodium items that they frequently used and were able to swap out a bunch.

My daughter is obsessed with all thing's beans, so she was happy to switch them out. Since the lower sodium cost her more, I just gave her all the cans we had as a fair trade.

My son loves pasta, so we told him which lower sodium pasta sauces, or no salt added tomato products. to get us and swapped all of ours with him.

We still had some things remaining which I held onto for times I would cook for non-CKD guests.

Yeah, it kind of sucked that I was preparing two dishes, one for everyone else and one for the hubby, but it was only temporary, until the stuff was used up.
Once it was used up, and still to this day, we make all CKD meals. Period.

We just tell everyone it is CKD and to salt up to their liking. Not a complaint yet!

I know… a lot of stuff here.
Read through, then let's head over to investigating.
Put on your cape and hat and grab your magnifying glass.

INVESTIGATING

All right let's discuss investigating.

I will do a ton of research online and I will go and check every grocery store within a 5-mile radius. And I have many.

- Checking ahead of time will also save you time in the store and cut down on reading all the labels.
- When I am in the store, I will still compare other items to the ones I have noted, simply because sometimes websites don't list all their products, or the info is out of date.
- Even when you do find a product that you like and you buy often, always double check the label. As mentioned before, manufacturers often will change their recipes.
- Each store will offer items that another store doesn't. This can be extremely frustrating because then you need to make several stops to get a hold of those items that work best for you.
  - When I find those ingredients, I will list them and the store that they are found at, so I have that for future reference. At some point you may run out and think oh where did I get that item from? If you have a list, you'll be able to look up right away where you got it.
- It usually happens that I must make a pickup order from Whole Foods and then shop at my nearest grocers for the remaining products. Yeah, kind of a pain sometimes but, at least we can create great tasting foods!
- When you must go to a different store for specific items, stock up while you're there so you don't have to return each time that you need it. If possible, just have it delivered.
- You can always check any specialty or ethnic stores in your area too. Many times, they will have products that are much better. Again, stock up so you don't need to return for a few months or more.
- Your local co-ops will have great produce plus many of their options are great. Think healthy store!

See, not too bad, right?

Just some great tips to help you out.

To continue helping you out, let's move over to the shopping unit where I can share all my great tips about that topic.

SHOPPING

All right, we touched on a little bit about shopping in our investigating unit so let's continue.

I still spend a lot of time in grocery stores and researching online. I am always on the lookout for better options and new ingredients or products that I can utilize to improve recipes and flavor.

- The more shopping you do, the more familiar you will become with name brand products that are acceptable and will purchase them often.
- The biggest thing is to have any reference sheets you may need with you or on your phone before heading out the door. Have that grocery list cheat sheet I created for you on your phone, so you have a quick reference sheet when choosing products.
- Make sure you have at least 1 or 2 alternatives listed on your grocery sheet for your fruits or veggies. If they are out or if you don't want to buy that bag of 6 turnips, you have an alternate ready.
- Make sure you plan your trips to cut down on the number of stops you will have to make.
  - Plan your big shopping trip which will include all non-perishables plus 3 days' worth of perishables.
  - Plan your next stop on day two or three for the remaining perishables for the week. This stop should be quick as most of it will be produce items.

BUDGETS

Let's talk about costs.

I know many people will get a little worried when the normal can of beans will cost between one and two dollars, but a can of low sodium may cost nearly twice that, or more.

- First thing, always look for the no salt added or low sodium store brand that will help to save money.
- Second, keep in mind that with CKD meals, the protein portion in your meal is often lower.
  - So that 1 pound of meat you used to buy for one meal is now two meals.
  - Often, we only use 1 cup out of those cans of beans, leaving 1/2 cup behind. If you want to save some money, use half the can of beans instead, and save the other half for another recipe. This helps to kind of balance out the differences in cost and you have slightly reduced some nutrients, that's ok!
    - Think of it like this: before, you were buying 1 pound of ground beef, 1 or 2 cans of beans, and probably a can of tomato sauce for your meal. Now, you will buy 1/2 pound or buy 1 pound and freeze the other half for another meal, and only 1 can of beans, and if you do buy tomato sauce, it will be a small 8 ounce can instead. You can see how that helps to even it out.
  - Now, if you really, really cannot afford anything but the absolute cheapest items because your budget is tight, get the store brand, and if the store brand doesn't have the no salt or low sodium options, go ahead, and buy it.
    - Just remember to rinse your beans and veggies extremely well to reduce that sodium by about 40% (as discussed in book one). Then reduce or omit the salt you would have normally added to your dish to keep sodium on the lower side.

- Third, check out the vegan and vegetarian options, maybe start incorporating more of them into your dish. Often, they can be less expensive than meat these days.

-
  - Speaking of this, you could reduce the amount of meat in your recipes to 1/4 pound and then supplement another 1/4 to 1/2 pound of a plant-based meat alternative into your dishes.
    - You can start using 1/4 pound of meat, and chop it small, in your meals. Now, 1 lb. of meat is going to work for 4 meals. Money saved.
  - Start making beans, grains, pasta, or low potassium veggies the star of your dish.
  - Here's a little tip... fat and fiber are the key ingredients to making you feel full. I hear a lot of people say that they do not feel full unless they have large portions of meat. If we need to reduce meat, then we can up the fat or fiber to replace it and make you feel full.

FINDING PRODUCTS

- Some other places to shop are the specialty food stores or ethnic grocers, as previously mentioned. They may carry hard to find items such as spices and condiments, and fruits.
- Check the organic and health food sections, especially for great produce.
- Check international or imported sections as previously mentioned as well.
  - They can contain a wealth of products that are much lower in sodium and with fewer preservatives than American products. They might be slightly more expensive but are worth it and often the items you are buying from these sections are products you use small amounts of.
    - For example, when I was looking for items like capers or olives, I could not find low sodium, but when I looked in the imported section, I was able to find those with much less sodium. To us, the extra cost was worth it as we were able to have these items in our meals. Plus, we still needed to use smaller amounts, so it lasted quite a while.
- I love to occasionally shop at World Market®. They carry a lot of imported products.
  - For those of you looking for a less sweet, less sugar treat, check the British snacks and desserts there. So yummy!
- If all else fails, shop online. I have listed some stores that carry exceptional products and usually list the nutritional information, so look at some of those.

When shopping, always start with the inner isles as you will spend more time reading labels.
Then grab your produce and then work your way around the perimeter and end at the cold and freezer sections.
From there, head to the register. I hope you can see how quickly that moves and how you cover the entire store. You keep cold things cold cos you are grabbing them right at the end and bagging them together will keep them cold until you get home.
I also love to play a great game of "Tetris" when I pack my bags too. We have a detached garage, so I like to have as few bags as possible to drag into the house, especially in winter.

Yes, I am one of those people you see with the bags draped on every arm, leg, waist, around my neck...

whatever it takes to get it into the house in one trip. It drives my hubby crazy. Although, this could maybe be a contributing factor to my need for shoulder surgery…

Anyways, I hope these tips help with your shopping adventures too.

Now, solidify that grocery list. Grab any reference sheets. Then place your order, pick it up, or go shop for your list.

Don't worry, this process gets to be second-hand as you become familiar with it. It really gets easier and quicker.

When ready, let's get cooking! And don't worry, the next section is quite easy.

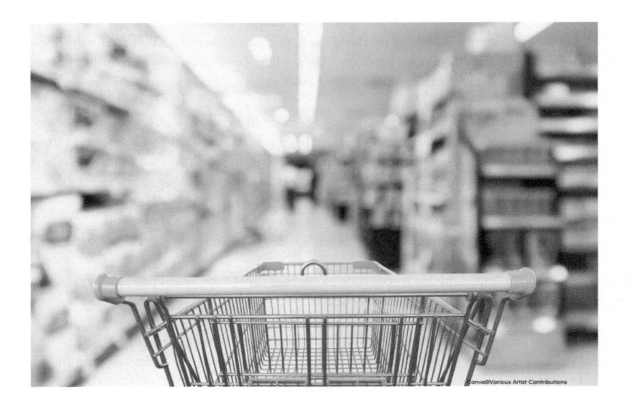

SHOPPING TIPS AND LINKS

- Have reference sheets with you or on your phone.

- Plan trips for big shops and remaining small shops.

  o Plan your big shop to include all non-perishables plus 3 days' worth of perishables.

  o Plan your next stop on day 2 or 3 for the remaining perishables.

- Shop the interior first as it will take most of your time reading labels.

- If possible, research everything online first. Then note the specific items on your list.

- Still check other items in store that may not have been listed online.

- 1 pound meat is often two meals. 10-12 ounces of alternative meats is often two meals.

- 1 can of beans, drained equals about 1 1/2 cups.

- If your recipe calls for an unavailable amount, go smaller. For example, 10 ounces of riced cauliflower often comes in 12 ounces frozen or an 8-ounce shelf stable cooked. If you choose the 8 ounces, your potassium is kept lower.

- Talk to your department heads at your grocers. Find out nutritional info if meats have been injected with solutions, baked goods' nutritional info, etc.

- Check all products that say low sodium. Many times, they aren't as low as their competitors.

- Check all store brands. Often, they are cheaper and nutritionally better.

- Check the organic and health food sections. Often have better options.

- Check the international or imported sections. Often have better options.

- Choose your meals based on leftover ingredients you need to use up or on foods you have in your pantry or freezer.

- Choose meals based on your weekly activities. If you know you are going to have a particularly busy week, plan simple meals or meals that can be done in a slow cooker or InstaPot® and set the timer so they can start on their own.

- Always look for sales or generic items first.

- Avoid the big displays and end of isle displays. Look at the top and bottom of the shelves as the less expensive items are often placed there.

- If shopping an order online, set pick up for after work. Picking up means you don't have to tip anyone.

- Early morning is the least busy time for shopping.

- Look for markdowns, especially meats. The expiration is coming soon, and stores slash the price to sell it quickly. You can freeze those items just fine.

- Stock up on sale items, especially meats. Vacuum seal if possible, and freeze.

- Buy frozen or canned vegetables, frozen fruits, dried beans, and rice. I

  o If you have a pressure cooker, beans and rice cook quickly.

- Use your pressure cooker/InstaPot® or slow cooker to cut down on time spent in the kitchen.
- Shop the bulk bins for items you only need a small amount of, like nuts and grains.
- Shop when you are not hungry or shop online, so you won't be tempted by impulse buys.
- Shop stores that sell produce items individually, like parsnips, carrots, turnips, zucchini, etc.
- Shop with a family member so you can share the costs and split up the food.
  - For example, a bag of carrots.

Shop these great places online…

ALDI'S https://www.aldi.us/

THRIVE MARKET https://thrivemarket.com/

HEALTHY HEART MARKET https://healthyheartmarket.com/

NETRITION https://www.netrition.com/

WORLD MARKET https://www.worldmarket.com/

OLIVE NATION https://www.olivenation.com/

TARGET https://www.target.com/

AMAZON https://www.amazon.com/

WHOLE FOODS https://www.wholefoodsmarket.com/

VITACOST https://www.vitacost.com/

IHERB https://www.iherb.com/

MISFITS MARKET https://www.misfitsmarket.com/

TRADER JOES https://www.traderjoes.com/home

VEGAN ESSENTIALS https://store.veganessentials.com

WALMART https://www.walmart.com/

SPICES INC. https://spicesinc.com/

LOV3 IT S3ASONINGS https://b-cindustries.com/

THE BRITISH DEPOT https://thebritishdepot.com/

FINDING ACCEPTABLE CKD PRODUCTS

Big chain stores carry so much more but don't always have what you need. Here are a few tips:

- Stores like World Market and Home Goods have great imported foods sections.

- Check out local stores in your area that you do not frequent. Perhaps Trader Joe's, Whole Foods, Aldi's, Fresh Thyme, and even Target can have some gems.

- Look for local ethic stores as you can find some great produce, seasonings and sometimes canned goods, legumes, grains, and condiments.

- Misfits Market, and Imperfect Foods are great options. They specialize in products that large chains reject due to their appearance.

- Ask your local grocer to carry items. One thing we LOVE but do struggle to get is Boar's Head low or no salt added cheeses and meats. We are talking about deli meats! Yes… roast beef sandwiches can be had. Sadly, you cannot order from their site, you must find a grocer or request that yours carry it. We only have two stores that carry limited items, and we must drive a bit to get to them but, when that craving hits for a grilled turkey and cheese sandwich, the drive is worth it!

- Have friends or family check some stores in their area and have them send it to you.

- You could look for restaurant supply stores too. The only drawback is that you will be buying in bulk…

- If you know someone with a Costco or Sam's Club membership, go with them and see what great items you can find. Ask if they are willing to split the item and the cost. If not, find a friend or neighbor that may be interested in splitting it with you.

- Do a general search online for what you are looking for. Do some research and when you find the best item, search that and see what websites (or stores in your area) carry it.

- There are amazing sites devoted to spices, baking supplies, imported foods, low sodium products, and more. Some of my favorites are Olive Nation, Healthy Heart Market, Spices Inc., British Essentials, British Food Depot.

- As always, Check Amazon. They seem to have nearly everything!

With some research and digging, you can usually find a great product. If you do need to order online, shipping costs (and delivery time) can be an issue. I would suggest buying a few of the item(s) you are looking for, so you have it on hand and do not have to place another order right away.

If all research and avenues let you down, and you cannot use an acceptable substitute, set that recipe aside and make it when you can get the product you need or make your own.

Making your own can be fun and rewarding. You may even find that you end up sticking with it, especially if it is an item that is frequently hard to get/find, or you realize how much more of it you can use because you made it yourself and lowered the sodium (or another nutrient).

There are options, you just need to become a bit of a detective to find them. Good luck!

Linda was the Chef for American Kidney Fund®'s Blog. A portion of this material was supplied to them on the blog. For more information, visit their site.

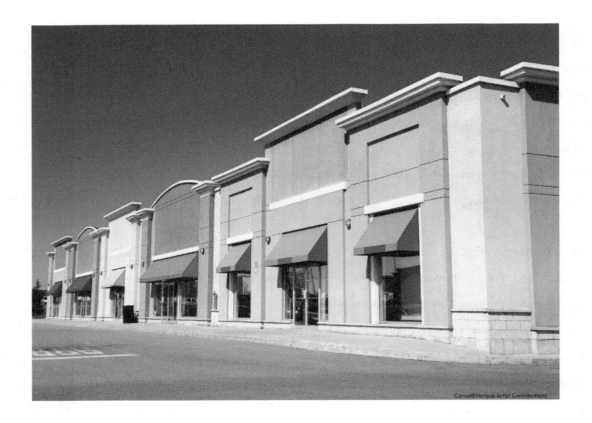

Canva©Various Artist Contributions

HOW TO CUT FOOD COSTS

We are all facing the rising costs of food and trying our best to keep expenses down but still eat healthily for CKD, right? There are ways to lower your costs and still eat for your kidney friendly diet. Here's a few tips.

MEAT
- Buy the cheapest cuts of meat and take advantage of sales. The trick to working with cheap cuts is to use the cooking method that is best for them. The easiest and best option is to toss them into a pressure cooker. This will help tenderize the meat. Alternatively, you can do a long, slow braise or place them in a slow cooker.
- Now is the time to shop with family and friends to buy large cuts of meat and share it. Portion it out into the amount you use most often, label, date, and freeze it.
- Go back to bone-in meats. Many of them are cheaper. Learn how to break down a chicken because, pound for pound, a full chicken is less expensive. You get 2 breasts, wings, legs, and thighs, plus a carcass that is great for making your own stock.
- Swap the meats in your recipe. Many times, you can swap the meat you are using and go with whatever is cheapest.
- Look for no salt added or lower sodium canned meats.
- Try vegan or plant-based meats as a whole or half replacement for your meat.

VEGETABLES & FRUITS
- Take advantage of sales on canned and frozen fruits and vegetables.
- If possible, grow your own vegetables and plan to can them this fall.

NUTS & BEANS
- Adding chopped nuts to dishes can help increase protein as well.
- Try adding 2 tablespoons or depending on other ingredients in your dish, up to 1/4 cup of chopped nuts.
- If you want to save money, you can buy dried beans. This way you can control the amount you use and if you have a pressure cooker, they can be cooked quite quickly. Dried beans are shelf-stable for a long time.

GRAINS
- Whole or refined, grains can help to add bulk to meals and thicken soups and stews. They can even be used in burgers and meatloaf to help retain moisture.

DAIRY
- Dairy products are becoming more expensive and there aren't a lot of alternatives to replace the creamy, rich products.
- Go for the cheapest and make a lot of substitutions when needed. If a recipe calls for yogurt and all you have is sour cream, use it.
- Do some investigation into non-dairy alternatives. Those babies have come a long way and many

products are great. The only exception is if you are a cheese snob. If so, get real cheese! I haven't found many vegan cheeses I like but, that's me.

I hope some of these tips will help you with your next shop and cooking!

Linda was the Chef for American Kidney Fund®'s Blog. A portion of this material was supplied to them on the blog. For more information, visit their site.

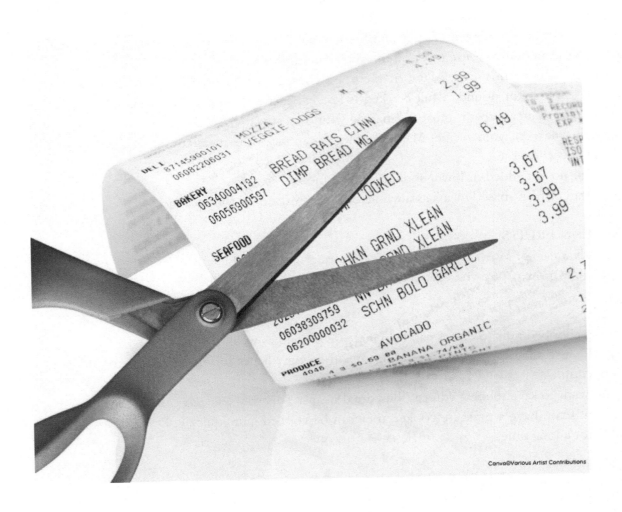

Canva@Various Artist Contributions

WHAT TO DO WHEN A FOOD ITEM IS OUT OF STOCK

Here are a few tips to help you navigate out-of-stock food and save money:

- Have one or two alternatives listed on your grocery list just in case the store is out of the food you were hoping to get.
- If you have your phone handy, do a quick search on Google for "best sub for [your item]."
- Read food labels to find one that closely matches the item you were originally looking for.
- Check the imported section or the health food section in your grocery store.
- Check to see if your item is available in canned, frozen, or pre-packaged version. If you end up with the standard, high sodium canned item, rinse it extremely well — which can reduce the sodium by nearly 40% - and omit or reduce any salt you would have normally added to your dish.
- If you purchase the higher sodium items, stick to the serving amount, or less.
- For stocks/broths, you can often use half the amount of stock, diluting it with water, to decrease the amount of sodium. Then add seasonings to help boost flavor; increasing the amount of each spice by one fourth in your dish will help keep flavors consistent and takes the guess work out of seasoning.
- If you need to substitute your usual meat option, look for low sodium or no salt added canned meats - they can work great in a pinch.
- For vegan meat-substitutes, be sure to double check the sodium, as plant-based meats are often high in sodium (and protein!).
- If you cannot find a substitute with similar nutrient levels, you can adjust your remaining meals for that day to compensate for the difference in that nutrient level in your meal plan. For example, if you end up buying a baked good that has higher sodium, reduce your sodium intake in your remaining meals that day.
- Order the food item online. Be sure to get a couple of them so you will have a supply if ever the food runs out again.
- Check for your ingredients at a different store. Just because your usual store is out, does not necessarily mean it is out at every store. Plan a trip to another one and see if they have your needed items in stock.
- Ask friends and family to keep a look out at their grocers for your items. If they find the items, have them purchase a few of them for you.
- For bakery items, condiments, sauces, stocks/broths and other similar items, plan to make your own if you know your grocer is often out of stock.
- Purchase meat in different forms to save some money. For example, if you purchase a roast or large chunk of meat, you can dice it yourself. You often end up with more than you need and can freeze the remaining for other meals. I do this often when I need beef stew meat. (Is it just me or is the cost of stew meat ridiculous?)
- It can be cheaper to buy boneless pork chops instead of a tenderloin, and hey, it is already cut up!
- If pre-formed hamburger patties are on sale, they can often be cheaper than ground beef.
- Preprocessed meats are more expensive, so purchase the bone-in pieces to save money. Plus, it adds more flavor to your dish.

- If you are purchasing vegan or vegetarian products, default to the basic ingredients and then add seasoning to better control the nutrients in the food. For example, instead of using the pre-seasoned tempeh "bacon," buy the plain tempeh and season it yourself. Look for plant-based meats in different forms. Often the pre-formed patties are less expensive than the crumbles.

Having a plan and being prepared is the best thing you can do to make kidney-friendly eating less stressful, especially when the food items you want are unavailable.

Linda was the Chef for American Kidney Fund®'s Blog. A portion of this material was supplied to them on the blog. For more information, visit their site.

<u>All the great tips I have shared in this section are listed out for your convenience, so you need not go searching. Ready?</u>

Organizing

- Whiteboard, dry erase markers, magnetic clips, calculator.

  o As mentioned, keeping a magnetic whiteboard, markers, and clips on your fridge will help you keep organized by noting items you run out of. Clips help hold your recipes. One for the recipes to be cooked, the other holds the ones that have been cooked. Always have a calculator handy for last-minute adjustments.

- Take inventory of leftover ingredients to use up. After making recipes you may have some leftovers like 1/2 cup beans, or some vegetables. Make note of those items and try to plan recipes that will help use them up.

  o Use veggies in quick breakfasts or lunches by making omelets, small salads, or make stock and freeze it.

  o Have a non-CKD person use them all together to make them into a soup and combine it with Italian sausage.

  o Create your own dish using them up on the weekend. Do some quick calculations of each leftover ingredient or simply have a "cheat day" and enjoy the Italian leftovers soup with your non-CKD person.

  o Freeze them or use fruits and veggies in compost or toss out for wildlife to eat.

- Do food/product swaps with family and friends.

Organize your shopping list by sections.

- Group them together by department. If possible, list those groups according to the layout of your store.

- Freeze leftover buttermilk, cream, half and half, egg yolks, and whites.

- Double the meals you cook and freeze for emergency days. Do this with any leftover portions too.

- Coordinate with sales when planning meals to save money.

- Work with family or friends to swap ingredients that you only need small amounts of.

Investigating

- Go online and find what stores have the items you need and begin a list of what products and where to buy them. You will always know where you got it and be able to make plans to shop.

- When you find a product that is the lowest or you really like, note it on your list. Even take a picture of it.

- Check products online ahead of time to cut down on some shopping time.

- Plan extra trips and orders for the items not at your main grocer and stock up so you only need to repeat this every few months.

- See if there are specialty or ethnic stores in your area. Check out the products they have. Again, stock up.

- Check for local co-ops. Many of their products are great and often, the produce is much better.

- Glance at the labels of the items you purchase often. It is common for manufacturers to change their recipes without notice.

Shopping

- Have reference sheets with you or on your phone.

- Plan trips for big shops and remaining small shops.

  o Plan your big shop to include all non-perishables plus 3 days' worth of perishables.

  o Plan your next stop on day 2 or 3 for the remaining perishables.

- Shop the interior first as it will take most of your time reading labels.

- If possible, research everything online first. Then note the specific items on your list.

- Still check other items in store that may not have been listed online.

- 1 pound meat is often two meals. 10-12 ounces of alternative meats is often two meals.

- 1 can of beans, drained equals about 1 1/2 cups.

- If your recipe calls for an unavailable amount, go smaller. For example, 10 ounces of riced cauliflower often comes in 12 ounces frozen or an 8-ounce shelf stable cooked. If you choose the 8 ounces, your potassium is kept lower.

- Talk to your department heads at your grocers. Find out nutritional info if meats have been injected with solutions, baked goods' nutritional info, etc.

- Check all products that say low sodium. Many times, they aren't as low as their competitors.

- Check all store brands. Often, they are cheaper and nutritionally better.

- Check the organic and health food sections. Often have better options.

- Check the international or imported sections. Often have better options.

- Choose your meals based on leftover ingredients you need to use up or on foods you have in your pantry or freezer.

- Choose meals based on your weekly activities. If you know you are going to have a particularly busy week, plan simple meals or meals that can be done in a slow cooker or InstaPot® and set the timer so they can start on their own.

- Always look for sales or generic items first.

- Avoid the big displays and end of isle displays. Look at the top and bottom of the shelves as the less expensive items are often placed there.

- If shopping an order online, set pick up for after work. Picking up means you don't have to tip anyone.

- Early morning is the least busy time for shopping.

- Look for markdowns, especially meats. The expiration is coming soon, and stores slash the price to sell it quickly. You can freeze those items just fine.

- Stock up on sale items, especially meats. Vacuum seal if possible, and freeze.

- Buy frozen or canned vegetables, frozen fruits, dried beans, and rice. I
  - f you have a pressure cooker, beans and rice cook quickly.
- Use your pressure cooker/InstaPot® or slow cooker to cut down on time spent in the kitchen.
- Shop the bulk bins for items you only need a small amount of, like nuts and grains.
- Shop when you are not hungry or shop online, so you won't be tempted by impulse buys.
- Shop stores that sell produce items individually, like parsnips, carrots, turnips, zucchini, etc.
- Shop with a family member so you can share the costs and split up the food.
  - For example, a bag of carrots.

Now that you've cleared all the topics from the board, let's head on over to spin the wheel and reveal your showcase!

9

Spin the Wheel & Head to the Showcase

You are rocking this.

As I had mentioned, this week's tasks are going to be very simple since you're going to be busy cooking. I have given you many reference sheets this week and all you need to do is look through them throughout the week and choose something from any of the sheets to try while cooking.

For example, look at your seasoning sheet and try toasting or blooming some of your spices. Or perhaps adding a splash of acid like lemon juice at the end of your dish.

Also, as a challenge try cooking one of your proteins to the correct temperature and letting it rest. Then taste it and notice the difference in taste, texture, and moisture compared to how you used to cook it.

That's it, that is all you must do this week!

Now please go through each unit, then implement any of the ones that really stand out to you. It could simply be improving the cooking method or correcting the temperature it tells you to cook the protein to. Maybe you have an idea for some seasonings to help improve flavor.

Just note any changes you make directly on your recipe so that way you can type it up so it's fresh and clean the next time you want to make it.

Then you can repeat the process of improving that recipe until you have it just how you like it. Type it up and keep it in a folder or binder as one of your go-to recipes.

The tips and tricks sheets are a big list of the many tips I have given throughout the course (this includes tips from book one). Some days it is easier to skim something like this than flip through pages.

When you are done with this week, we can start to celebrate! I will bring the balloons!

SEASONING (like a pro!)

Welcome to the unit on seasoning.
Here you are going to learn ways to season your meals that will bring about the best flavor.
You also get helpful information on subbing out seasoning.

Sometimes you only have dried spices or herbs instead of fresh ones and you need to know how much you can use.
That information is here.

I also share a few tips about salt alternatives.

I've included a handy little list of common seasonings and their amounts. For example, if your recipe calls for 1 teaspoon of caraway seeds this will let you know that the equivalent is three-quarter teaspoon ground. I've come upon this situation many times so I know how helpful it can be.

The key points to seasoning are to allow them enough time to release their flavor, which is 20 minutes minimum, when, and how to use them, and learning the process of layering them.

When I say layering, this is what I mean.
The flavors you want as the undertone of the dish should be added early. This allows the flavor to get into every nook and cranny of the meal.
Think of those meditation audios and how they always have some music or a hum in the background that is constant. You hear it and know it is there, but more attention is paid to other sounds, like chimes, bells, birds, etc... That background or hum is the first layer of seasoning.

The seasonings that you want to be the sounds, are added midway through cooking. These will impart flavors but won't have quite the depth and continuous hum as the first ones. You may pick up on their flavors more quickly or be able to identify them.
This could be something like the ocean sounds that sit just above that background hum.

The seasonings you add right at the end or as a garnish are the prominent, hit your tongue, you can taste them flavors. Think of the fresh and bright flavor pop the parsley garnish gives.
This is the equivalent of those bells or birds in the meditation audios. They are the forward sounds.

As you can tell by this explanation, I see, hear, and think things quite differently.
I warned you; I am a weirdo!
But I am betting 100% that you now understand layer!

Keep this info handy the next time you are cooking.

SEASONING FOR BEST FLAVORS

When to add seasonings depends on what you are using

- Dried or ground spices and herbs need heat, fat or liquid and a minimum of 20 minutes to release their flavors.

- Fresh, delicate herbs should be added right at the end for a bright burst of flavor. Basil, chives, cilantro, dill, mint, parsley, tarragon. Most delicate herbs do not have woody stems.

- Fresh, robust herbs can be added early. Bay leaves, marjoram, oregano, rosemary, sage, thyme.
  - Most robust herbs have woody stems, and you will usually add the sprigs to the dish and will need to remove them before serving.

General Rule for Subbing

- if the recipe calls for dried and you want to use fresh, use 3 times the amount and add at the correct time.

- If using dried instead of fresh, add the dried with the other seasonings in the dish.
  - 1 teaspoon dried = 1 tablespoon fresh. 1 tablespoon fresh = 1 teaspoon dried.

- If the recipe calls for dried and you have ground, use about 1/3 the amount. 1 teaspoon dried = 1/3 (think heaping 1/4) teaspoon ground.
  - For example: subbing ground thyme for dried thyme leaves.

Blooming

- You can bloom your dried spices and seasoning to bring their flavors forward.
  - To do this, when you have melted your fat, add the spices and cook briefly, 10-15 seconds. Do not bloom pungent spices or that will become the overriding flavor in your dish.

Toasting

- You can bring extra flavor by toasting the dried seeds such as cumin, coriander, etc.
  - Place them into a dry skillet over medium-low heat and toast them until they begin to darken. Stir or shake frequently so they do not burn and become bitter.

Layering Flavors

- The seasoning flavors you want as the undertone of the dish should be added early. This allows the flavor to get into every nook and cranny of the dish. Think of those meditation videos and how they always have some music or a hum in the background that is constant. You hear it and know it is there, but more attention is paid to other sounds, like chimes, bells, birds, etc... That background or hum is the first layer of seasoning.

- The seasonings that you want to be the sounds, are added midway through cooking. These will impart flavors but won't have quite the depth and continuous hum as the first ones. You may pick up on their flavors more quickly.

- The spices you add at the very end, or the herbs you use as a garnish are like a big clang of cymbals. You notice them right away, above all else.

- **Tip**! rub seasoning into the meat or add with the sauces for best flavor distribution.

Acid is a great alternative to salt.

- Citrus juices and vinegar can be added right at the end of a dish or squeezed on top when serving. This tricks the tongue into believing it tastes salt.

Switch to kosher (coarse grain) salt, like Morton's.

- Coarse grain salt needs to dissolve in liquids to avoid big bites of salt.

- Teaspoon for teaspoon, it contains less sodium than regular table salt.

- When making a dish, add it to the liquids right away so it has some time to dissolve.

- For baking, crush or grind first or add it to the liquids instead of the dry ingredients. Stir it frequently to help it dissolve faster. You can use the full amount called for in the recipe. Baked goods are usually divided into numerous amounts (36 cookies, 12 pieces of cake….) which means the resulting amount of sodium per serving will be small.

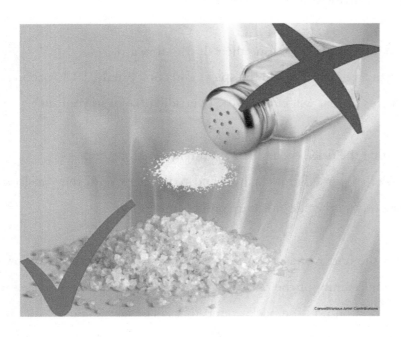

HELPFUL SEASONING INFORMATION

- Achiote / Annatto: 1 1/2 teaspoon seeds = 1 teaspoon ground
- Anise: 1 star = 1/2 teaspoon seeds, 1/4 teaspoon ground
- Bay leaf: 1 fresh = 2 dried leaves, 1/2 teaspoon ground
- Caraway seeds: 1 teaspoon seeds = 3/4 teaspoon ground
- Cardamom: 10 pods = 1 teaspoon, 1/2 teaspoon seeds, 1/2 teaspoon ground
- Celery seeds: 1 teaspoon seed = 1 teaspoon ground
- Chili Peppers: 1 fresh or dried = 1 teaspoon ground
- Cinnamon: 3-inch stick = 1 teaspoon ground
- Cumin seeds: 1 teaspoon seeds = 3/4 teaspoon ground
- Cloves: 1 teaspoon whole = 1 teaspoon ground
- Coriander seeds: 1 teaspoon seeds = 1/2 teaspoon ground
- Dill seeds: 1 teaspoon seeds = 1 teaspoon ground
- Fennel seeds: 1 teaspoon seeds = 3/4 teaspoon ground
- Garlic: 1 large clove = 1 tsp minced, 1/4 tsp powder
- Garlic: 1 small clove = 1/2 tsp minced, 1/8 tsp powder
- Garlic salt: 1 teaspoon = 1/8 teaspoon garlic powder plus 1/16 teaspoon salt
- Ginger: 1-inch = 1 tablespoon grated, chopped, or minced; 1/4 teaspoon powdered
- Juniper berries: 1 teaspoon berries, 3/4 teaspoon ground
- Mustard seeds: 1 teaspoon seeds, 1 teaspoon ground
- Onion: 1 medium fresh (1 cup) = 3 tablespoons dehydrated chopped, 2 tablespoons dehydrated minced, 1 tablespoon powder or granulated
- Onion: 1/2 medium fresh (1/2 cup) = 1 1/2 tablespoons dehydrated chopped, 1 tablespoon dehydrated minced, 1 1/2 teaspoons powder or granulated
- Onion: 1/4 medium fresh (1/4 cup) = 3/4 tablespoon dehydrated chopped, 1/2 tablespoon dehydrated minced, 3/4 teaspoon powder or granulated
- Peppercorns: 1 teaspoon peppercorns = 1 teaspoon ground
- Turmeric: 4-inch = 1 tablespoon grated, chopped, or minced, 1 teaspoon ground

Fresh herbs are difficult to measure as the sizes can vary greatly. Measure for accuracy.

Fresh herbs: 1 tablespoon chopped = 1 teaspoon dried = 1/4 teaspoon ground.

These are all the herbs I was able to find info for.

- Anise (star): 1 star = 2g
- Basil: 1 medium leaf = 1/2g
- Bay leaf: 1 fresh = 1/2g, 1 dried = 0.6g
- Chives: 1 tsp chopped = 1g
- Cilantro: 1 medium sprig = about 2g
- Dill: 1 medium sprig = about 0.2g
- Epazote: 1 sprig = 2g
- Kaffir lime leaves: 1 leaf = 1g
- Mint: 1 medium leaf = 0.05g
- Oregano: 1 sprig = 2g
- Parsley: 1 medium sprig = 1g
- Rosemary: 1 sprig = 2g
- Saffron: big pinch = 1g
- Sage: 1 medium leaf = 1g
- Tarragon: 1 sprig = 2g
- Thyme: 1 sprig = 1g

COOKING TEMPERATURES

All right let's talk about cooking temperatures and a few tips.
I have seen countless recipes telling people to cook their proteins to horrific temperatures.
Seriously, if you cook a chicken breast too long, you're not going to be able to chew it!
You might be able to use it as a baseball, but you're not going to eat it.

So here I am giving you the correct temperatures to cook foods that will result in the best textures and flavors and still be moist.

The key to keeping your proteins moist is to let them rest.

I said let them rest.

I'm sure you've heard this a million times before, but it is very important.
- Think of it like this: when you boil a vegetable, what happens? It floats to the top and jumps around in the bubbling water. When you turn off the heat, it eventually settles back to the bottom.
- This is like meat. When it is hot, all those juices come bubbling up and party on the surface. If you don't let that rest, you will lose all that moisture.
- When you rest it, all those juices are going to stop partying and go home, back inside the meat. When you have rested it, then cut it into it, it will be beautifully juicy.

When at a restaurant, I can always tell if they have rested the meat or not.
If the plate comes out with a ton of red-hued liquid all over and running into my potatoes, I know it came straight from the pan.
I don't want the drippings in my potatoes. Yay for hot food but, who gets their food and thinks well darn, I need to wait a few minutes to let this rest?
Nobody. You dig in.

I always take note of such crazy little things.

Now with bigger proteins like a roast or a turkey, you are going to let them rest much longer.
For those everyday things like hamburgers or steaks or pork chops you only need to let them rest for three to five minutes.
It's not like you are waiting forever!

So read through this information and if needed, write it up and slap it on your fridge using one of your magnetic clips, and have it available so you always know what temp to cook those proteins to.

I think you can tell that this is clearly a pet peeve of mine.
Hey, we spend a lot of money on food, it should taste good!

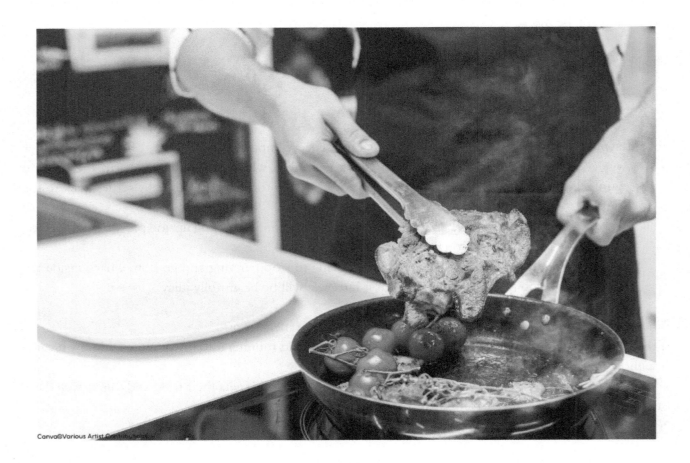

Canva@Various Artist Contributions

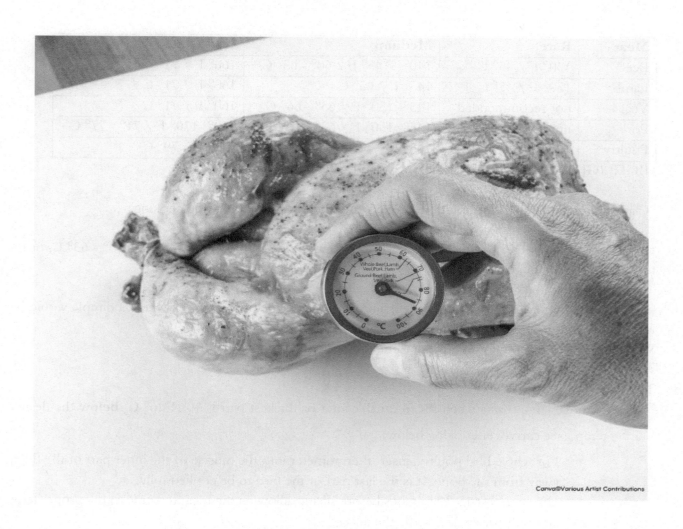

Canva©Various Artist Contributions

FOOD TEMPS

Food	Safe Temp
Plant based / Fruit / Veggies / Grains / Beans	135° F / 57° C
Steak / Chops / Fish / Seafood*	145° F / 63° C
Ground Meat / Eggs	165° F / 74° C

Meat	Rare	Medium	Well Done
Beef	130° F / 45° C	140° - 145° F / 60° - 63° C	160° F / 71° C
Lamb	130° F / 45° C	145° F / 63° C	160° F / 71° C
Veal	not recommended	145°- 150° F / 63° - 66° C	160° F / 71° C
Pork	not recommended	145°- 150° F / 63° - 66° C	160° -170° F / 71° - 77° C
Poultry*	not recommended	165° F / 74° C	175° F / 79° C

HIGHLIGHTED BOXES ARE THE "SWEET SPOT".

*Clams, Oysters, & Mussels should be cooked until their shells open during cooking.

*Wild duck, Pheasant, & Quail should be cooked to a <u>lower</u> temp of 140° 145° F / 60° - 63° C, or the meat will become tough and dry.

RARE: soft, gives to pressure but not jelly-like. Touch the side of your cheek where a dimple would be.
MEDIUM: moderately firm, springs back readily. Touch your chin.
WELL-DONE: firm, does not give in to pressure. Touch the tip of your nose.

TIPS!
- Remove large roasts when the internal/center or thickest part is 10° F (6° C) **below** the desired temp. (see carryover cooking below)
    - For whole bird poultry, insert thermometer into the muscle of the inner part of the thigh, away from the bone. It is the last part of the bird to be cooked fully.
    - Let them rest 15-30 minutes before slicing, allowing the meat to come to the proper temp and redistribute and settle the juices.
    - Let smaller meats, like chops and breasts rest for 3-5 minutes.
- Carryover cooking can raise internal temperatures from 5°F (3°C) for small cuts to as much as 25°F (14°C) for very large roasts and birds.
- **THE DANGER ZONE! 41°—135°F (5°—58°C).** Foods left at these temperatures run the risk of rapidly growing bacteria, causing several illnesses. Also, do not leave food sitting out for more than 2 hours.

COOKING METHODS

Welcome to Cooking Methods!
In addition to cooking temps, cooking methods are just as important. They can create so many wonderful flavors.

Think of the difference between a grilled chicken breast and one that was baked.

Many times, recipes will tell you to blanch or deep fry or to braise, or pan broil etc.
You may not know what those terms actually mean, which means you don't actually know how to cook it the way they say to.

So, I listed them as a guide to tell you about each method.
There may be some you're not familiar with, this way you can learn what they are, and this will also help with cooking your meals and producing better results.

Keep in mind that some terms we use here in America do not mean the same as they do in other countries. If you are in another country, read through, and have a giggle at our differences.

COOKING METHODS GUIDE

Please note that these are U.S. terms and some of them mean different things in different countries.

- **Bake** – dry heat cooking in an enclosed space, usually an oven. Can also be done in hot ashes or on hot stones. Bread, pastries, fish, vegetables, dough, batters.

- **BBQ** – a low and slow, smoke roasting technique using a wood fire, in a pit. This is often now referred to when grilling or smoking. Most often used for large pieces of meat.

- **Blanch** – a food is dipped in boiling water or boiled for up to 2 minutes, then plunged into ice water. This stops the enzymatic actions that cause loss of flavor, color, and texture. This allows you to delay cooking or to freeze. Vegetables and fruit.

- **Boil** – cook in rapidly bubbling liquid. 212° F / 100° C. Grains, pasta, pulses, eggs, vegetables, meat.

- **Braise** – cook, covered, in a small amount of liquid, usually 1/3 to 1/2 the way up the side of the meat. The meat is often seared first. Braising liquid is frequently used to make sauces. 200° - 300° F / 94° - 150° C. Large and/or tough cuts of meat, vegetables.

- **Broil** – rapid, high, heat from above. 500° - 550° F/ 260° - 289° C. Lean, thin cuts meat, vegetables, fish, browning or melting.

- **Deep Fry** – submerging food in hot fat. Typically, 350° - 425° F / 177° - 218° C. Breaded or battered are common. Meat, vegetables, dough, drop batters.

- **Drying / Dehydrating** – low humidity, low heat, with plenty of air circulation. If living in an appropriate climate, sun drying is an option. Air drying is done indoors in well-ventilated areas. Often used to preserve foods. Use of an appliance or can be done in the oven. Lean meats, fruit, vegetables.

- **Griddling** – heat from below, on a solid surface, using little if any fat. Typically, around 350° - 375° F / 177° - 191° C. meats, vegetables, sandwiches, eggs, pancakes.

- **Grilling** - heat from below, over open grid. Temperature is controlled by moving foods from direct heat to indirect heat. Many grills allow you to control the temperature settings. Low heat: 300° - 350° F / 149° - 177° C., Medium heat: 350° - 375° F / 177° - 191° C., Medium-high heat: 375° - 400° F / 191° - 204° C., High heat: 450° - 600° F / 232° - 316° C.

- **Microwave** – use of an appliance ranging in wattage from 500 to 2,000. Cooks outer edges first. Uneven cooking. Overcooking occurs often. Food often dries out. Will not break down connective tissue. Will not produce tender meat. Best for reheating, thawing, frozen meals, quick melting or softening. Do not use metal.

- **Pan Broil** – no fat added, or liquid used. If fat accumulates, pour it off so it does not fry in it. Cooked in a fry pan or skillet, uncovered, and usually preheated. Nonstick pans work best. Thin cuts of meat or fish.

- **Pan Fry** – moderate amount of fat used (more than used when sautéing), longer cooking time, moderate heat. Best for small portions of food. Food is flipped, not tossed. Larger pieces of meat like chops and chicken.

- **Parboil** – partial boiling. Boil food for a short amount of time. Similar to blanching but cooking for a slightly longer time and is not plunged into an ice bath. Food will be reheated or finished cooking at a later time. Meat, vegetables, nuts, fruit, grains, beans.

- **Poach** – cook in a liquid that is hot, but not bubbling. 160° - 185° F / 71° - 85° C. Eggs, meat.

- **Pressure Cooking** – utilizing an appliance or special pot. Cooking under high pressure steam. Tenderizes meats very well and in less time. Often foods are placed under a broiler or in a hot oven afterwards to brown them. Almost anything can be cooked in a pressure cooker.

- **Roast** – uncovered, no water used. Heat cooks the food evenly on all sides. Temps range from 300° - 500° F / 149° -260° C. For browning, drying, or parching. Meat, vegetables, nuts.

- **Sauté** – quick cooking time, in a small amount of fat, over high heat. Food is often tossed, not flipped. Vegetables, thin or small cuts of meat.

- **Searing** – over high heat, cooking the surface of the food on both sides until a browned crust forms. Use a high smoke point oil. Meat is usually finished cooking in the oven. Optionally, heat is reduced and cooking finishes in the pan. Meat.

- **Simmer** – cook in a liquid that is bubbling gently. 185° - 200° F / 85° - 94° C. Covered or uncovered. A slower and gentler cook. Grains, beans, vegetables, meat, fish, stock.

- **Slow Cooking** – utilizing a slow cooker or crock pot appliance. Used as a convenient sub for braising. Keep temperatures low, around 210° for at least an hour, to break down connective tissue and render fat. Most anything can be cooked in a slow cooker.

- **Smoking** – cooking, browning, flavoring, or preserving foods by exposing it to smoke from burning wood. Meat, fruits, vegetables, cheese, nuts, eggs, seafood.

- **Sous Vide** – vacuum sealing food in a bag or jar and cooking in a water bath at a precise temperature. Meat is often seared after cooking to add browning and flavor. Requires special equipment. Meat, fish, seafood, vegetables.

- **Steam** – cook by exposing food to steam, above boiling water or in steam cookers. Retains more nutrients and color than boiling. Takes longer. Fish, vegetables, meat, seafood, eggs, dough, fruits.

- **Stewing** – like braising but for smaller items. Often using more liquid. May or may not be seared first. Long and slow cooking. Think stew and chili.
- **Stir Frying** - fried in a small amount of very hot oil, over high heat, while being stirred or tossed in a wok. Vegetables, thin cuts of meats or alternative proteins, sometimes grains or noodles.
- **Tagine** - use of a specific cooking vessel (tagine), usually ceramic or clay. Covered with the lid, food is cooked over a smoldering charcoal fire. For stove, use a diffuser and cook over a medium-low heat for long periods.
- **Toasting** – browning with direct dry heat. Use of an appliance is common. Can toast nuts and seeds in a skillet or in the oven. Usually done in a short amount of time.

FOOD STORAGE

Welcome to this section on food storage.

When working with CKD meals it's often the case that you were going to have leftover ingredients.

- For example, when you're only using one quarter to a half a pound of meat, you're going to have the other portions left over.
- If you're using half a can of beans or half a can of vegetables, you will have the other half left over.

So here, in this unit, I give suggestions that you can use to store your food so that it will last a little bit longer.

I have also given you information on some safety tips such as temperatures that food should be stored at, and food placement.

- For example, the location of foods in your fridge does make a difference.

- **_Very Important!_** When you are thawing meat, or keeping it in the fridge, you should <u>always</u> have it in a high sided pan to avoid any leaking and contamination of other items in the fridge.
- **_Never_** leave meat sitting on the counter to thaw.

I have also given you some information on the various fruits and vegetables that should or should not be refrigerated.

So have a look at all this great information and if you need to, go ahead, and rearrange that fridge.

When you're finished rearranging the fridge, I will see you in the next one.

STORING YOUR FOOD

Freezing

- Set your freezer to 0° F/ -18° C or lower. Set your fridge below 41° F/ 5° C.

- Get yourself some good, airtight storage containers and freezer safe containers.

- Use your dry erase marker to write on your containers when placing them in the fridge.

    o Mark the contents and the date. The dry erase will wash off.

- Alternatively, have freezer tape and a permanent marker to label the frozen items with the contents and date.

- If you use freezer safe disposable bags, you can use the permanent marker to write on the bag.

- How long you keep the leftovers is up to you. Some people won't eat leftovers, others will eat them after a week. Generally recommended to eat the next day but never go beyond two or three days.

- Frozen foods should be kept for three to six months.

Food Placement

- Practice FIFA (first in, first out). Do this with all food products. When you buy something new, place it in the back so the next item you take is the one that will expire the soonest. That way you are using up products before they expire and not throwing any away.

- Do not overcrowd your fridge. The air needs to circulate properly. If a product isn't getting enough cold air, it will spoil sooner.

- Only buy 2-3 days' worth of perishables at a time. If you know you won't have the opportunity to shop in a few days, then buy a few more days and store those items in the very back of the correct drawer. It is colder there and will help keep them longer, especially herbs and greens.

-

    o **Top** shelf of the fridge should hold ready to eat items, leftovers, drinks, herbs, some condiments that are not acid based or stored in brine.

        ▪ This area holds a consistent temp.

    o **Middle** shelf should contain cheese, eggs, cooked meats, tortillas, pitas, wraps, and breads. You can store bread in the fridge, but it will dry it out. If I know we won't be using it quickly, I fridge it.

        ▪ This area holds a consistent temp also.

    o **Bottom** shelf should contain dairy products, raw or thawing meats which should be in a pan to catch any liquids that may leak. This helps avoid cross contamination. Some fridges now have drawers specifically for meat.

- The back of the bottom shelf is the coldest spot in the fridge.
- **Crisper drawers** hold the vegetables and fruits. Many fridges have separate drawers for fruits and vegetables.
- **Door shelves** should hold nonperishables, condiments, dressings, and acidic foods or those in brine.
  - This is the warmest spot in the fridge.

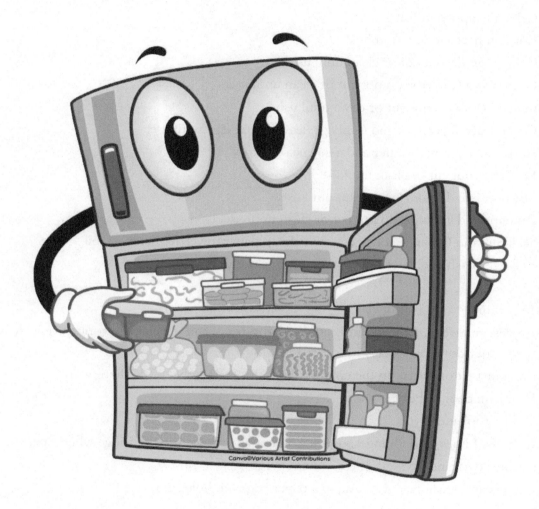

TO FRIDGE OR NOT TO FRIDGE. THAT IS THE QUESTION...

Refrigerated

- Asparagus: in a cup with 1-2 inches of water.
- Bell peppers and Hot peppers: do not cut or clean until use.
- Berries: do not cut or clean until use.
- Broccoli and Cauliflower: do not cut or clean until use.
- Carrots: baby carrots or cut carrots are wrapped in, or covered with damp paper towels, changed often. Full carrots should remain in their bag. Do not cut or clean until use.
- Celery: wrapped in foil.
- Corn: in package or left in husks.
- Cucumber: do not cut or clean until use.
- Grapes and Cherries: do not cut or clean until use.
- Green beans: do not cut or clean until use.
- Green leafy vegetables and Cabbage: leave in package until use.
- Herbs: in a cup with water and a baggie over top.
- Leeks: do not cut or clean until use.
- Mushrooms: do not clean or cut until use.
- Parsnips and Turnips: do not cut or clean until use.
- Scallions and Green onions: wrap in a damp paper towel and wrap in foil.
- Yellow squash and Zucchini: do not cut or clean until use.

Not Refrigerated

- Apples: release gases that cause other nearby fruits and vegetables to ripen quickly. Give them space, they don't play well with others.
- Basil: in a jar of water, on the counter. Yep, this is the rebel of the herb world.
- Eggplant: cool and dry.
- Garlic: cool and dry.
- Lemons, Limes, and Oranges: on the counter and move into the fridge when ripe.
- Melons: cool and dry.
- Onions and Shallots: cold, dark, in a paper bag with holes in it.
- Squash: cool and dry.
- Stone Fruits (any fruit with a seed inside): on the counter and move into the fridge when ripe.
- Tomatoes: cool and dry, move into the fridge when ripe.

KITCHEN GADGETS

Welcome to Kitchen Gadgets!
In this unit I want to let you know of some helpful kitchen gadgets.
All these things are extremely useful in the CKD Kitchen.

Because that simple little ingredient, salt, is kept to a minimum, we must utilize a lot of different tricks to keep flavor in our meals.
To do that there are some gadgets that are extremely helpful.
Do not feel that you must go out and buy all these things, they are merely suggestions.

- **#1** super strongly suggest you get a digital thermometer. For safety reasons I always, always temp my meat to make sure it is properly cooked.

- **#2** is the food scale. This is the second item I super strongly suggest you get. I use mine daily, for anything and everything, not just when baking. I have several scales and all of them have at least an ounce setting and a gram setting.

These below are super great but get 'em only if'n ya want to. (Somehow, playful doesn't come across well in print. Ha!)

- Another great tool is the micro plane grater. I used to use my cheese grater because I was stubborn and didn't see a reason to change. Then it broke and I decided I would just get the micro plane. I am telling you it was like day and night. The micro plane is amazing at zesting spices and citrus. It results in a much finer zest.

- There is an item also listed on here that you may or may not be familiar with called the Frywall® splatter guard (search Amazon). To be honest I hate to fry food. Without fail I always get splashed with some pop of grease from the pan and burned. I swear I hear giggling from the pan too! This fry wall will sit inside of your pan and help to reduce those chances and catch a lot of the grease that would normally fly out all over your stove, your counter, or on you. It is a little bit tricky to measure for the right size. I kept measuring wrong and actually ended up with all three sizes before I got it right. But I still love using it.

- I am going to give you a little tip and that is… nonstick pans really aren't needed except for delicate items like eggs, pancakes, or crepes. I own one nonstick pan just for that purpose. There is still a lot of debate about the possible toxicity of non-stick cookware.

- Sometimes we may want to impart some flavors from our seasonings, but we don't want to add any ground seasonings. This is especially true if we are making a stock. In those cases, is a great idea to use a sachet or mesh tea bag to hold those larger items like cinnamon sticks and whole cloves or whole allspice berries and star anise etc. Using one of these will prevent you from having to fish them out afterward.

- And lastly, I will mention the mini mortar and pestle. I do have a spice grinder which I will use for bigger amounts like a spice blend. But I will use the mortar and pestle for smaller amounts, especially when I need to grind my kosher salt up into finer crystals, usually for baking. Super quick, super handy.

Again, don't feel you need to buy any of these. You may have done perfectly well all this time without any of them.

I find they simply help make things easier.

KITCHEN GADGET INFORMATION

These items will help make meal preparations easier and faster, allow for more accurate portions and may involve less clean-up.

- **Calculators** will come in handy when you are reducing or doubling a recipe, or when you need to divide a dough into several equal portions. Or when calculating amounts of sodium per serving in a dish.

- **Digital thermometers** are used to make sure your food is cooked to the right temperature. No overcooking, no under-cooking. Not only can you check meats and vegetables, but you can check the temperature of baked goods as well (baked goods are considered cooked at 200° F / 94° C).

- **Dry erase markers** are constantly utilized in my kitchen. You can write directly on your container lid, and it will wash off. I purchase the markers with magnets and keep them on my fridge (turned upside down so ink is fresh).

- **Dry erase white board** is highly recommended. Get one with magnets on it and place it in the fridge. Anytime you run out of an ingredient, list it right away. This will always keep you up to date and shorten the time you take to make your grocery list. Get a large one for listing freezer contents too; you can erase an item when you pull it out of the freezer, and you can always see what you have on hand to work with or use up!

- **Extra measuring spoons and cups** for solids will be used daily and it helps to have several on hand, especially when baking or when making dishes with many measurable ingredients.

- **Extra measuring cups** for liquids because liquids measure differently than solids. For accuracy, make sure you are using the right ones. (Look for the glass cups).
  - I highly suggest you buy two, 1-cup, and one of each of the 2 cups and 4 cups.

- **Fine mesh strainers** in various sizes **or cheesecloth**. A small strainer is great for sifting small amounts or when sifting powdered sugar over a dessert. Larger sizes work perfectly when you need to strain tiny sized pasta or sauces with small herbs you want to filter out. I also use cheesecloth on occasion when making dishes that require moisture to be squeezed out such as cucumbers and spinach. Cheesecloth can be washed or simply tossed.

- **Food processors** are a great tool to have. I suggest getting a small one, like a mini-Ninja®, and a large one, if possible. Many dishes require processing small amounts, and nobody wants to pull out the large processor just for that. A food processor will not give you a smooth sauce, however. A blender will work best for that. Yes, I have a mini blender too.

- **Food scale** with both ounces and grams. This is the second most used item in my kitchen. When portioning meats or weighing ingredients for baked goods, it helps create a better dish and allows for more accurate portions.

- **Mandolin and/or Spiralizer** are great at slicing items thin, or long, or in noodle forms. This is perfect for salads or when subbing veggie noodles (flat or thin) in your dish.

- **Microplane** graters are amazing at zesting citrus and spices. These produce a much finer zest than using a cheese grater.

- **Mixer attachments** are available for some countertop mixers. They can peel, rice, spiralize, create vegetable or pasta sheets, grind meat, and more.

- **Cheese graters** are an option if you want to save money. Buying blocks gives you more cheese for your money. Plus, blocks do not contain anti-caking agents. But… you must take the time to grate and then wash the grater.

- **Citrus Juicers/Squeezers** are perfect to bring those bright and fresh zingy flavors and to replace salt. The handheld citrus squeezer is great for smaller citrus like lemons and limes, the manual juicer works best for larger citrus, like oranges.

- **The Frywall® Splatter Guard** is wonderful if you detest the raining of grease over everything while you are frying. The trickiest part is finding the size that is right for your pan. Start midway up the side of the pan, on the inside, and measure across to the other side. This is where the guard will sit in the pan as you fry. (Seriously, look it up on Amazon!)

- **Nonstick pans** are perfect for delicate items such as eggs, pancakes, crepes, or toasting spices.

- **Small saucepans** are perfect for small sauces. Again, no need to pull out a large pan for such a small amount. I own two and yes, I have used them both at the same time.

- **Sachet bags or mesh tea bags** are perfect for placing fresh herbs and spices into your dish. Plus, easy removal at the end. No more stirring and fishing around for that stray bay leaf, the twig of thyme, or that star anise. There are also silicone herb infusers as well, so you are not throwing away any bags.

- **Spice grinder or mini mortar and pestle** are perfect when you have toasted your spices and want to grind them or when you are baking, you can use the mini mortar to crush the kosher salt into a fine texture. Less sodium is added but in smaller grain form for better incorporation.

- Twine: kitchen twine is available and useful for tying up meat and sachet bags.
  - **Tip!** When using a sachet bag, cut an extra-long piece. Tie the bag and tie the other end to the handle of your pot. No fishing around when you want to remove it!

WEIGHTS & MEASURES

How many times have you been in the kitchen and needed to make an adjustment? Needed to know a specific measurement or convert from one unit to another?

Don't fret! Here I have supplied you with weights and measurements info.
I've tried to think of every possible area I struggled with regarding weights and measurements.

I have listed out a lot of different things here that could help you.
When cooking or working through recipe adaptations, you can grab your calculator and do some quick converting, if needed.

You are doing so well.
Can you believe how far you have come?
You can start to see how working the method is going to finally give you the ease you've craved for so long.

Linda Blaylock

WEIGHTS & MEASURES

Weights & Measures

1 teaspoon = 5 ml
1/2 oz = 1 tablespoon or 3 teaspoons or 15 ml
1 oz = 1/8 cup or 2 tablespoons or 6 teaspoons or 30 ml
2 oz = 1/4 cup or 4 tablespoons or 12 teaspoons or 59 ml
2 2/3 oz = 1/3 cup or 5 tablespoons plus 1 teaspoon or 16 teaspoons or 79 ml
4 oz = 1/2 cup or 8 tablespoons or 24 teaspoons or 118 ml
5 3/4 oz = 2/3 cup or 10 tablespoons plus 2 teaspoons or 32 teaspoons or 158 ml
6 oz = 3/4 cup or 12 tablespoons or 177 ml
8 oz = 1 cup or 16 tablespoons or 237 ml

Basics

1 tablespoon = 3 teaspoons
2 tablespoons = 1/8 cup or 6 teaspoons
3 tablespoons = 9 teaspoons
1/4 cup = 4 tablespoons or 12 teaspoons
1/3 cup = 5 tablespoons plus 1 teaspoon or 16 teaspoons
1/2 cup = 8 tablespoons
2/3 cup = 10 tablespoons plus 2 teaspoons
3/4 cup = 12 tablespoons
1 cup = 16 tablespoons

4 ounces = 1/4 pound
8 ounces = 1/2 pound
12 ounces = 3/4 pound
16 ounces = 1 pound
20 ounces = 1 1/4 pounds
24 ounces = 1 1/2 pounds
28 ounces = 1 3/4 pounds
32 ounces = 2 pounds

If recipe calls for instant yeast, and you only have active yeast, multiply by 1.5.
Example: recipe says 2 teaspoons instant
2 tsp x 1.5 = 3 teaspoons of active needed.

Now reverse it. If recipe calls for active and you only have instant, divide by 1.5.
Example: recipe says 2 teaspoons active
2tsp / 1.5 = 1.34 teaspoons of instant needed.

Grams and milliliters are more dependable. Weights will vary by ingredient.
Example: 1/4 cup of flour is 40g, while 1/4 cup sugar is 60g.

Common Weights of Teaspoons

Baking powder 4g
Butter 4.5g
Flour 2.6g
Gelatin 3.6g
Instant yeast 3g
Oil 4.5g
Salt (table) 6g
Salt (kosher, coarse) 3g
Sugar (granulated) 4.2g
Sugar (powdered) 2.8g
Sugar (brown) 4g
Swerve (granular) 4g
Vinegar 4.79g
Water 4.93g

©2022 CKD Culinary Consulting. All Rights Reserved

122

WEIGHTS & MEASURES

Liquids

1 oz = 30 ml

2 oz = 59 ml

3 oz = 89 ml

4 oz = 118 ml

5 oz = 148 ml

6 oz = 177 ml

7 oz = 207 ml

8 oz = 237 ml

9 oz = 266 ml

10 oz = 296 ml

11 oz = 325 ml

12 oz =355 ml

16 oz = 473 ml

Oven Temps

Cool Oven: 170° – 200° F / 77° – 94° C

Very Slow Oven: 200° – 250° F / 94° – 121° C

Slow Oven: 250° – 325° F / 121° – 163° C

Moderately Slow Oven: 325° – 350° F / 163° – 177° C

Moderate Oven: 350° – 375° F / 177° – 191° C

Moderately Hot Oven: 375° – 400° F / 191° – 204° C

Hot Oven: 400° – 450° F / 204° – 232° C

Fast or Very Hot Oven: 450° – 500° F / 232° – 260 C

Convert Inches to Centimeters

1 inch = 2.54 centimeters

divide cm by 2.54 = inches

multiply inches by 2.54 = cm

Convert Celsius to Fahrenheit

Celsius divided by 0.56 = X

X + 32 = F

Milliliters to ounces: ml divided by 29.6

Ounces to ml: Multiply ounces by 29.6

Pounds to ounces: Multiply pounds by 16

Ounces to pounds: Divide ounces by 16

Cups to ounces: Multiply cups by 8

Ounces to cups: Divide ounces by 8

Pints to ounces: Multiply pints by 16

Ounces to pints: Divided ounces by 16

Quarts to ounces: Multiply quarts by 32

Ounces to quarts: Divide ounces by 32

Common F to C Temps

F		C
140°	=	60°
145°	=	63°
160°	=	71°
165°	=	74°
170°	=	77°
175°	=	79°
180°	=	82°
200°	=	94°
220°	=	104°
225°	=	107°
250°	=	121°
275°	=	135°
300°	=	149°
325°	=	163°
350°	=	177°
375°	=	191°
400°	=	204°
425°	=	218°
450°	=	232°
475°	=	246°
500°	=	260°
525°	=	274°
550°	=	288°

Dash
1/8 teaspoon or 0.62 ml

Pinch
1/16 teaspoon or 0.31 ml

Smidge or grain
1/32 teaspoon or 0.15 ml

Sugar Work

	F	C	
Thread:	230°	110°	(syrups, some icings, liqueurs)
Soft ball:	240°	115°	(fondant, fudge, caramels, meringues)
Firm ball:	245°	118°	(caramels, butter creams, toffee)
Hard ball:	250°-260°	122°-127°	(caramels, nougat, divinity)
Small crack:	265°-270°	130°-132°	(butterscotch, taffy)
Hard crack:	290°-310°	143°-155°	(glazed fruit, brittles, spun sugar)
Caramel:	320°-340°	160°-170°	(molds, pralines, brittles)

CKD Culinary Consulting

THE BIG LIST OF HELPFUL TIPS

HANDY DANDY TIPS!

This is a **large** collection of many of the tips that may have been mentioned throughout the course. Yes, this includes those tips from book one as well!

Sometimes it's much easier to be able to skim over something like this than it is to go back and dig through pages and books or try to read any notes you may have scribbled down.

Just one more way that I am trying to make things as easy as possible for you.

Tips & Tricks

Before cooking, measure out all ingredients first. This will alert you if you have run out of something. This also allows your cooking process to go much quicker with everything in hand. I will often line items up on the counter in the order they will be added to the dish as well.

MEATS
- Dice, mince, shred, chop, puree ingredients for better distribution.
- Choose cheaper cuts of meat for braised or stewed dishes. The longer cooking times will tenderize the meat and it will save you money. Using a pressure cooker will reduce cooking time and create tender meat.
- Always use a thermometer to check the temperature of your meat.
- Cut meat against the grain for a more tender bite. Look at the side of this piece of beef. See how the grain or lines are running lengthwise?

**If you cut in the same direction as the grain, your meat will be tough.
If you cut across/against the grain, you are breaking up the meat fibers which yields a more tender bite.**

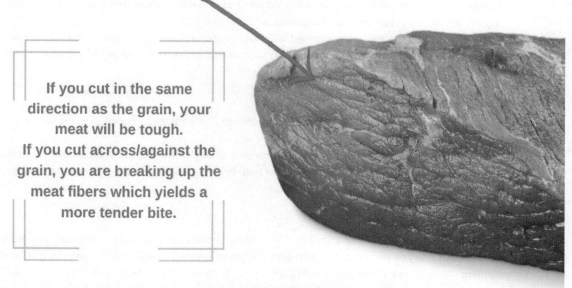

- When cooking bacon, always add it to a cold pan. Heating the pan and bacon together will render more fat. This works with precooked bacon as well.
- Look for a statement like "retained water solution" or "mechanically tenderized" on packaged and frozen meats. Look for the smallest amount available. Read that statement as "we injected potassium, and/or phosphorus, and more than likely, sodium into this product and we aren't going to tell you how much".
  - Look for celery or rosemary preservatives on ground meats for your best option.
- Recipes calling for ground beef will be 80-85% lean, unless specified.
- Refined oils are best for high temps and frying. Unrefined and virgin oils are best for low heat or dressings.
- Use panko soaked in stock for moist meatloaf. "the moist-maker" some of you will get that reference.

Tips & Tricks

FRUITS & VEGGIES

- Dice, mince, shred, chop, puree ingredients for better distribution. Yes, I will forever drill this into your brain! When chopping veggies for a meal, chop extra for the next meal so you have them ready.
- Include a 1/4 cup side of fruit with your meal to add a healthy side dish, get more fruit in your diet, and it often eliminates the need for a dessert.
- Swapping riced or spiralized veggies in a dish works well but can leave your dish watery as they do not absorb the liquids. If subbing, reduce the liquids in your dish by 1/4 to 1/2 cup, sometimes more.
- For wonderful flavor, roast your garlic. Cut off the top, drizzle with oil and wrap in foil. Place in the oven for 30 minutes at 400°F / 204°C. You may remove cloves from the bulb and place them in foil instead.
- To easily peel a garlic clove, lay it on your cutting board and with your hand, a small dish, or cup, or side of your knife, press down on the clove until you hear a crack. Then peel.
- Dialyze your root vegetables. Remember that piece of info way back in unit 1? Double boil your root veggies to remove almost 50% of the potassium. Yay!
- Frozen, fresh, canned, etc. using canned will usually result in lower potassium. Look for no salt added. If you cannot find that, look for lower sodium and make sure to drain and rinse to remove up to as much as 40% sodium.

NUTS & SEEDS

- If you wish to add nuts or seeds to your recipe, limit to 2 tablespoons chopped unless you know the specific nutritional info of the recipe.
- When you open a new jar of nut butter and the oil is sitting at the top, get your electric hand mixer and use the dough hook attachment. This will help mix everything and save you a sore arm. Hang on to that jar!!

DAIRY

- Use strong flavored and sharp cheeses. If you cannot have a lot of cheese, make sure you taste it.
- Temper your dairy or mix each cup with 2 teaspoons of a starch before adding to your dish to avoid curdling. Dairy does not like high heat (180°F / 82°C or more). Always best to add it at the end.
- More fat in dairy equals less phosphorus, and lower chance of curdling.
- You can freeze cream, buttermilk, half and half, egg yolks, egg whites, fresh herbs in oil, etc. Freeze them and keep a running list of what you have.

EGGS

- Egg shell and yolk colors due not indicate better nutrition. It only tells you what colored hen it came from and what they ate.
- Red spots? Ok. Whites are greenish? Ok.
- Egg whites are pink or pearl? Toss. Black or green spots? Toss.
- Float in water? Toss.
- Stands up at the bottom? Use soon, hard boil them now!
- Not floating or standing in water? It's fresh.

Tips & Tricks

BEANS & GRAINS

- Combine incomplete proteins to form a complete protein. Remember... rice and beans!
- Remember to get enough fiber. Men 30g or more and women 21g or more per day. Don't overdo it or you could be faced with some uncomfortable GI issues.
- If you cannot find low sodium or no salt beans, make sure to rinse them thoroughly before using. This will reduce up to 40% of the sodium.

PASTA

- Cooking time on boxes of pasta is too long. Begin checking it 5 minutes before the box says it should be done. Pasta should have a slight bite to it.
- Use 2 ounces of dry pasta per person.

VEGAN & VEGETARIAN

- Note the plant or bean used as the base of the product to gauge nutrition.
- You will often have to stick to the serving size.
- Use a basic item like tofu or tempeh instead of processed or seasoned.

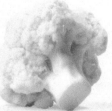

NON-DAIRY

- Use non dairy alternatives in high dairy recipes to lower phosphorus.
- Coconut milk in recipes refers to the canned unless specifically stated to use the drinking.

GLUTEN FREE

- Gluten free mixes should be mixed longer and should rest for at least 10 minutes or more. This will build strength and allows the starches to absorb the liquids. Yes, complete opposite of gluten flours.
- Gluten free bakes also take longer to cook and brown quickly. Increase baking time and reduce the oven temp by 25°F / -4°C.
- Gluten free has some seriously tasty treats. Goodie Girl®, Enjoy Life®, Schar® to name a few.
- Use 2 tablespoons of gluten free breadcrumbs in 1/4 cup of broth to add to meatloaf.
- Cook gluten free noodles longer. Remove earlier and/or rinse in cold water to stop the carryover cooking.
- Do not combine noodles with the dish until serving. Store leftover separately.

LOWER CARB

- LowER carb meals will give you more flexibility than strict low carb meals.
- Avoid any and all protein powders, if possible.
- Check fiber amounts, they can be high.
- You can use more than cauliflower and zucchini.

Tips & Tricks

CONDIMENTS
- Look for vegan alternatives, many times the sodium is much lower.
- Make your own. (see unit 4 for the DIY sauces and seasoning recipes)

FATS & OILS
- Refer to your reference sheets for high smoke point oils and proper storage.
- If unsure, use olive oil.

ALCOHOL & SUBS
- If using a vinegar or citrus juice to replace alcohol, dilute it first.
- Look for the alcohol free extracts. See the website suggestion in module four spices.
- Never, ever buy crappy "cooking wines". Buy a cheaper wine to cook with and save the more expensive wines for drinking.
- Make sure you cook your dish for a long enough period to evaporate the alcohol. 30 minutes = 35% remaining. 1 hour = 25% remaining. 2 hours = 10% remaining. 2 1/2 hours = 5% remaining. 3 hours, good to go.

SPICES
- Use woody stemmed herbs early in your dish. You can also add them to the fat in the beginning.
- Add delicate (non woody stemmed) herbs at the end or as a garnish.

NATURAL SWEETENERS
- Sugar helps to balance flavors, especially acidic and bitter flavors.
- It also helps balance flavors in dishes with high amounts of fiber.
- Adds bulk in baking.
- Sugar helps prevent bacterial growth. Think of it as a natural preservative.
- It weakens gluten and makes baked goods soft, and frozen products smooth, in addition to adding volume, strength, and fluffiness.
- It helps with creaming. When the amount of fat in a recipe is half the amount of the flour or more (by weight) you want to cream the fat and sugar. This adds air into the mix. The sugar jumps in and breaks apart the fat to make room for the air. This helps create a rich and fluffy texture.
- It caramelizes well. This aids in the beautiful browning of baked goods and sauces.
- It's one of yeast's favorite foods!
- Look for Brer Rabbit® mild molasses. Best found so far in regard to potassium.

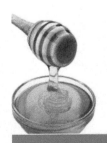

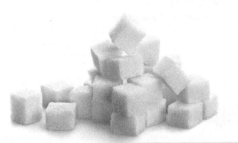

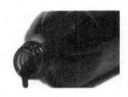

Tips & Tricks

ALTERNATIVE SWEETENERS
- Alternative sweeteners tend to be even sweeter than sugar.
- Some work well with cold ingredients while others will not.
- Some work well with high temps, others will not.
- Does not add bulk, often less browning, no rise, drier products and must adjust oven temps and times.
- Many have aftertastes ranging from metallic to cooling to numbing.
- All can cause gastrointestinal issues if consumed in excess.
- Combine two or more sweeteners to help mitigate the aftertastes and produce better products.
- Our bodies digest half of the sugar alcohol content.
- Total carbs – fiber + 1/2 of the sugar alcohols = true net carb count.

FLOURS
- You can toast flours at any temperature in the 300°F to 400°F / 149°C to 204°C range.
  - Preheat the oven to the temperature for your recipe. Once preheated, place the sheet pan into the oven and allow the flour to toast, stirring once halfway through. Or you can cook it over medium to medium-low-heat on the stove, whisking constantly. For a medium toast, cook for about six to seven minutes. For a dark toast, cook for about ten minutes.

ALTERNATIVE FLOURS
- Lower your oven temperature by 25°F or –4°C. And bake it for a longer amount of time.
- Find your favorite items and stick with them. If you use a different product, it can change how the recipe works.
- Always try to stick to something similar. If you are out of almond flour, sub with another nut flour. If you are out of a starch, sub with another starch.
- Let batters and dough rest for at least 10 minutes, 30 would be better.
- Beat the batters and dough more.
- Let bakes cool in pans or on the sheets to firm up.

THICKENERS, BINDERS, GUMS, LEAVENERS
- Always make a slurry for thickening.
- Some thickeners create a gelatinous texture.
- Cornstarch does not like acidic ingredients, Arrowroot is not as happy with dairy.
- Do NOT add more, let the dish cool to reveal the true thickness. Remember my arrowroot story?
- Try to stick to 1 teaspoon of baking soda or powder.
- Baking soda needs an acid to activate it.

LABELS
- Look for "phos" on labels.
- Look for "retained solutions" in meats.
- Look for potassium chloride listed on lower or no salt products as a salt replacer and avoid it!

Tips & Tricks

PLANNING
- Choose your meals based on leftover ingredients you need to use up or on foods you have in your pantry or freezer.
- Choose meals based on your week activities. If you know you are going to have a particularly busy week, plan simple meals or meals that can be done in a slow cooker or InstaPot® and set the timer so they can start on their own.
- Use the FIFA method. First In, First Out. Rotate your foods, placing new purchases in the back and moving the older purchases forward to you use them first.

GROCERY LIST
- Group products together on your list. If possible, create list to match the store layout.

ADAPTING
- Look at the nutrient you are over in. Begin reducing or replacing those first.
- Continue to the next highest item containing that nutrient, reduce or replace, if needed.
- Add bulk back into your meals.

ORGANIZING
- Check your whiteboard for needed items.

INVESTIGATING
- Investigate products online first.
- Buy hard to find products online.

SHOPPING
- Double check labels routinely in case manufacturers changed their formulas.
- Stock up on items you buy at specialty shops to reduce the number of times you have to return there.
- Always look at store brands, generic items, and sales, first.
- If your protein is quite costly and no sale this week, choose a vegan or vegetarian option.
- Check the international, health food, vegan, low carb, and gluten free sections for more options.
- Many organic products are lower sodium.
- Avoid the big displays and end of isle displays. Look at the top and bottom of the shelves as the less expensive items are often placed there.
- If shopping an order online, set pick up for after work. Picking up means you don't have to tip anyone.
- Early morning is the least busy time for shopping.
- Look for markdowns, especially meats. The expiration is coming soon and stores slash the price to sell it quickly. You can freeze those items just fine.
- Stock up on sale items, especially meats. Vacuum seal if possible, and freeze.

Tips & Tricks

- Shop the bulk bins for items you only need a small amount of, like nuts and grains.
- Shop when you are not hungry or shop online so you won't be tempted by impulse buys.
- Shop stores that sell produce items individually, like parsnips, carrots, turnips, zucchini, etc.
- Shop with a family member so you can share the costs and split up the foods. For example, a bag of carrots.
- Shop inner isle first, then the perimeter.
- Shop your non perishables and 3 days of perishables first. Return on day two or three for remaining.
- Make sure you have reference sheets with you and some alternatives listed on your sheet in case they are out.

SEASONING

- If your dish is too bitter, sour, or salty, add sweet.
- If your dish is too sweet, add sour, bitter, or salty.
- If your dish is too spicy, add dairy. Never add salt as it will boost the spicy.
- If using nuts or seeds, (including seed spices like cumin or coriander seeds) toast them for 1-2 minutes in a dry skillet over medium-low heat. Keep the pan moving so they do not burn! You may grind them after, if desired. This will lend a nutty or toasty layer of flavor.
- Bloom (bring flavors forward or outward) mild seasonings with fat. Cumin or caraway seed, celery seeds, coriander seeds, and dried herbs are examples that benefit from blooming.
- Fat carries flavor and is a great option for blooming spices. Think infused butter.
- Do not bloom pungent or powdered seasonings like cayenne, cloves, allspice, pepper, or paprika in a dry pan, they will burn and / or become the dominant, overwhelming flavor.
- Add powdered seasonings with a carrier like fats or liquids.
- Dried or ground seasonings need a minimum of 20 minutes of heat to release their flavor.
- Layer your flavors. Remember the background hum and the sounds I had mentioned in the seasoning lesson in module nine?
- You can also rub spices into meat or toss with vegetables.

SALT

- Add an acid at the end of your dish before serving to replace salt. 1-2 tablespoons of lemon or lime juice is perfect. Or serve with a lime or lemon wedge to squeeze over top.
- Check out the great salt replacers. Mrs. Dash® line, Benson's® table tasty, True Lime/Lemon® line, and Orrington Farms® low sodium beef and chicken broth powders.

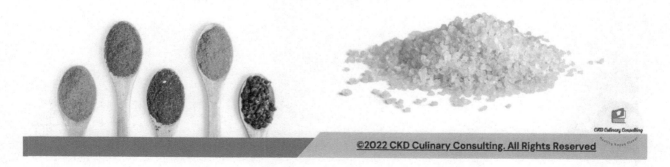

CKD Culinary Consulting

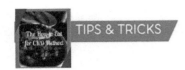

Tips & Tricks

COOKING TIPS

- Bulk up a meal with lower potassium vegetables, rice, pasta, couscous, orzo, or lower phosphorus beans like garbanzos.
- Dual cooking methods increase flavor. Roast vegetables before adding to the dish, sear meat before dicing and adding to the meal or braising.
- Low and long simmers help create flavors. Add ingredients at the right time, meaning, start by adding ingredients that take longer to cook and let them simmer for a bit. Next, add ingredients such as softer vegetables that don't take as long to cook, and let simmer again.
- Sweat your aromatics like onions, celery, carrots, and peppers at the start to release their juices and add flavor. Sweating means to cook them over a medium heat until they release their juices and soften. You will not be browning them. Note: garlic will burn easily. Best to add toward the end of sweating and only cook for 15 seconds to 1 minute.
- Heat your pan for a few minutes to prep the surface of it. Then add your oil and heat that for a minute. If oil is not hot, your food can become greasy. The exception is non-stick pans. Never heat them dry as they will emit toxic fumes. Always heat the fat with the non-stick pan.
- Do not use acidic ingredients like tomatoes, citrus, and vinegar in aluminum pans. The reaction can cause a bitter and/or metallic taste in your dish. Think about the tin-like or metallic taste of canned tomatoes. Ick.
- Use refined or hulled grains when using as a thickener. The bran/outer hull will not allow absorption of liquids.
- Use your pressure cooker/InstaPot® or slow cooker to cut down on time spent in the kitchen.
- Buy frozen or canned vegetables, frozen fruits, dried beans and rice. If you have a pressure cooker, beans and rice cook quickly.
- When grilling, it is best to start the meat over direct heat to get the wonderfully tasty char. Then move it over to indirect heat (not over the flames), to finish cooking.

Food Storage

- Label and date all leftovers and leftover ingredients.
- Do not crowd your fridge. Keep foods in optimal locations in your fridge.
- Set fridge below 41°F / 5°C, and your freezer below 0°F /-18°C.
- ALWAYS store meats in a high sided pan in the fridge to avoid contamination from leakage.

Gadgets

- A food scale works for everything. Get one with ounces and grams.
- Try the Frywall® splatter guard for frying.
- Use mesh tea bags for large spices and a microplane grater for fine citrus zest and spices.
- Use a mini mortar and pestle for grinding up small amounts of seasonings or your kosher salt.

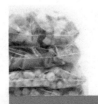

Tips & Tricks

BAKING

- Flour should always be scooped with a spoon into your measuring cup. Do not pack it down. If you simply scoop from the container, you can end up with too much flour and that can affect your bake.
- Always sift your flour.
- When relying on the reaction between an acid and baking soda for a fluffy rise, wait to combine the wet and dry ingredients until you are ready to place into the baking pan and bake right away.
- When stirring anything, do a figure eight motion. This will mix things more quickly and evenly.
- When pouring a batter into muffin liners, pans, etc, hold a spoon over top of the pan and allow the batter to pour onto the spoon and into the pan. This helps avoid splashes and hard plops which can release air. You can also use this same method when adding sauces into your savory dish.
- Never grease angel food cake pans. Make sure to cool them upside down.
- Grease the bottom of the pan only, for low fat bakes.
- If your recipe is high in fat (weight of the fat is the same or higher than the weight of the flour), it is best to start by creaming your fat with your sugar to whip some air into it. Then alternate adding the liquids and flour.
- If your recipe is low in fat (weight of the fat is less than the weight of the flour) but has plenty of eggs and sugar, this means they are depending on air for the rise. Whip your whites.
- Store yeast below 34°F / 1°C to keep it inactive.
- Yeast growth is best between 70°F and 90°F / 21°C and 32°C. Yeast dies at 140°F / 60°C.
- Dough should double in size. First prove is fine to collapse in on itself.
- Poke up to your second knuckle into the proved dough, if it remains indented, it is ready to shape.
- If it is contracting, rest it longer.
- If second prove collapses, rework, reshape, rise again.
- Never rise more than three times.
- Your dough is ready to bake when you poke a finger into it and it springs back.

REMEMBER!

- Remember! Our bodies absorb 100% of the phosphorus additives in foods. 80% from animal based dairy products, 60% from Meat, Legumes, and Nuts, and 40% from grains.
- Try some non dairy items. Try some vegan and vegetarian protein options. Expand your food options!

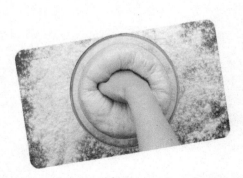 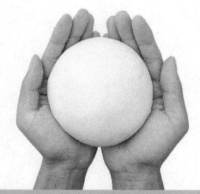

10

Congratulations!
You're the Grand Prize Winner!

You won!

Not only the completion of the program but you've gained a solid foundation for you to continue forward. Even better, you can take the already wonderfully tasty recipes of mine and you can adapt them. You learned it, you earned it.

Just grab your laminated sheet and use any other reference materials you need. These are your new best friends.

I am so proud of you and excited for you.

You now know how to eat for CKD and have full control over your diet.

Please continue repeating modules seven and eight.

You will find that portions of it will become extremely familiar and ingrained in your brain so that you will not have to strictly follow a sheet through the process.

It will become second nature to you and this process will speed up exponentially.

I hope that all the information I have given to you is quite helpful and has made this entire process very easy. Ok, easier…

I hope you were able to use a lot of my tips for cooking as well. Simply changing your cooking method will improve the flavors of your meals quite a bit.

This way you won't have to use your piece of chicken as a baseball, and you can actually eat it.

So, let's wrap all of this up.

There are several bonus recipe bundles coming up.

There is a barbecue bundle for those lovely summer days.

A gluten-free bundle with some of my favorite gluten-free treats.

A vegan and vegetarian bundle which, if you haven't tried these products yet, please do, they are quite tasty.

A lower carb bundle which may not be strictly low carb but are lower carb and of course are tasty.

And then I've given you a holiday bundle containing a bunch of different side dishes and a few desserts too. Give them a try.

Then more information for holidays, dining out, gatherings, or on the go and what to do in those situations.

And now I beg you please, please, be so kind as to submit the super quick evaluation feedback form.

It helps tremendously for others to read your thoughts and feelings and to take your recommendations.

Go here: https://forms.gle/rhKwWv7iiuzoGTWS6

If you would like to leave a review on Google,
please do so here: https://g.page/r/CYcRRI4GfFteEB0/review

If you want to jump over to Yelp and look me up there under "How to Eat for CKD", I would appreciate it a ton! I will even give you an extra balloon :-)

I would really love to hear what you think and how you feel about this program.

And finally, my heartfelt thank you is coming up.
Please continue being a part of the client Facebook group family (if you had chosen to do so) so I can continue to help and support you and to celebrate your wins too!

Let's get the party started!
(Cue balloon drop and music)

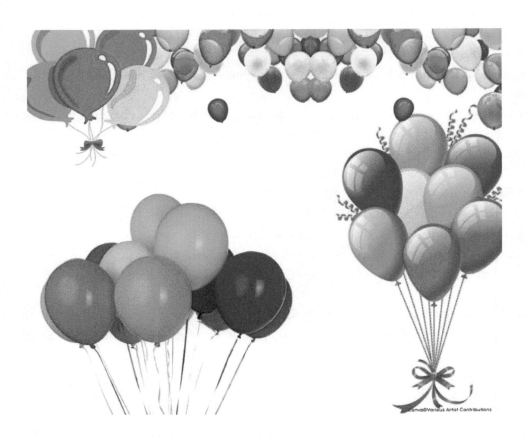

RECIPE BUNDLES

Here it comes!!

Several bundles of my favorite recipes just for you.

Please note that although the recipes may be lower in carbs, gluten free, etc.

<u>YOU CAN NOW ADAPT THEM!!</u>

You learned it, feel free to do it.

Many of the recipes are lower carb, gluten free, nondairy, etc. even though they are not within that bundle. This is a recipe that may have been created for that alternative diet but, it turned out so well, that it was kept and added to a bundle.

Again, feel free to use my suggestions to flip the recipes whenever the suggestions are offered.

If you want to try the recipe as is, that's great. You may find you love it as is.

For the salt lovers in your family, let them put a few sprinkles and they are going to enjoy it too.

Let's Eat!

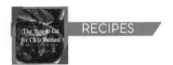

BBQ Recipes

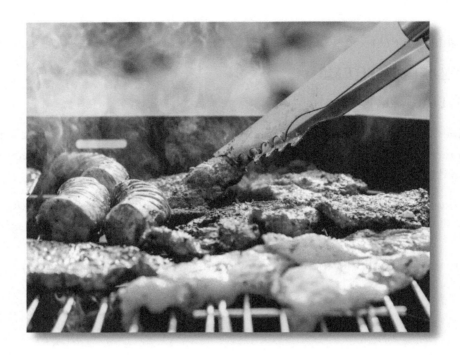

Creamy Mac & Cheese

Potato Salad

Sunshine Salad

Mojito Fruit Salad

No Bake Biscoff® Cookies

Banana Cream Dessert

Recipe: mac n cheese

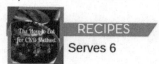

RECIPES

Serves 6

Creamy Mac & Cheese

Ingredients:

10 ounces large or 12 ounces medium elbow macaroni noodles, dry
30 grams Cheez-it® cheddar crackers (27 crackers)
1/4 cup panko breadcrumbs

SAUCE
1/2 cup heavy cream
1 large egg
2 cups water
1 tablespoon lime juice
1 tablespoon low sodium Worcestershire sauce
2 tablespoons unsalted butter
2 tablespoons flour
2 ounces cream cheese, softened
1 teaspoon ground mustard
1/2 teaspoon white pepper
1/2 teaspoon ground nutmeg
1/2 teaspoon kosher coarse salt
1/4 teaspoon paprika
1/2 cup shredded sharp cheddar cheese
1/2 cup nutritional yeast flakes

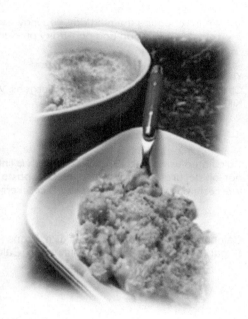

Instructions:

1. Preheat oven to 350° F / 177° C If baking. (See options in step nine)
2. Cook noodles according to package. If done early, toss with 2 teaspoons oil to prevent clumping.
3. Blend the crackers and panko in a food processor until small bits remain. Set aside.
4. For the sauce:
   a. Mix the cream and egg together.
   b. Mix the water, lime juice, and Worcestershire together.
   c. In a saucepan over medium heat, melt the butter. When melted, whisk in the flour, and cook about 2 minutes or until sand-like consistency.
   d. Add the cream cheese and all seasonings, whisk constantly until melted.
   e. Add the egg/cream mix and the water mixture. Whisk and cook until it starts to thicken.
   f. Add the cheddar and whisk until melted.
   g. Remove from heat and stir in the yeast.
5. Place half the noodles into a greased baking dish. Pour half the sauce over top. Place the remaining noodles in the dish and top with the remaining sauce.
6. Cover and bake for 20 minutes.
   a. If pressed for time, simply mix the sauce and noodles together with the cracker/panko mix and serve.
7. Remove from oven, place the cracker/panko mix over top.
   a. If desired, broil for about one minute. Watch it, as it will brown **very** quickly.
8. Divide into six portions and serve.

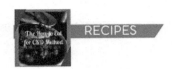

Creamy Mac & Cheese

Recipe tips:
- Suggest serving with 1/4 cup sliced strawberries, or lingonberries or a mix. Topped with a sprinkle of chopped basil per person.
- When reheating the next day, you may need to add a splash of oil.
- You may use vegan and non-dairy products to reduce phosphorus and fat.

Allergens:
Yeast, Dairy, Cheese, Eggs.
Check Soy and Worcestershire for allergens. Wheat/Gluten, Milk, Soy in Cheez It®. Wheat/Gluten, Yeast in Kikkoman® panko.

Nutrition Information:
Calculated using the NB2O system which is linked to the USDA database. Not lab tested so nutrition is not lab accurate. Calculated using 12oz pasta, Kikkoman® panko breadcrumbs, Kikkoman® Worcestershire sauce and Cheez It® crackers.

Calories: 466, Fat: 21g, Sat. Fat: 12g, Trans Fat: 0g, Cholesterol: 89mg, Carbohydrates: 53g, Fiber: 3g, Sugar: 3g, Sodium: 365mg, Protein: 16g, Calcium: 133mg, Phosphorus: 239mg, Potassium: 308mg

Recipe: potato salad

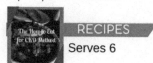

Serves 6

Potato Salad

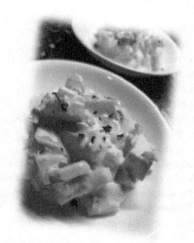

Ingredients:
3/4 cup mayonnaise
1 teaspoon garlic powder (if not a garlic fan, reduce to
1/4-1/2 teaspoon)
1/2 tablespoon sugar
1 1/2 tablespoons apple cider vinegar
2 teaspoons Dijon mustard
1 1/2 cups baby red potatoes (4-6, depending on size)
2 tablespoons red bell pepper, chopped
1/4 cup onion, chopped
1/4 cup celery, chopped
2 large eggs, hard boiled and chopped

Instructions:
1. Mix the mayonnaise, garlic powder, sugar, vinegar, and mustard together. Set aside.
2. Chop the potatoes and boil until tender but still firm. Timing will depend on the size of your cuts. There should be a bit of resistance when poked with a fork.
3. Drain the potatoes and rinse them under cold water until they have cooled. Set aside.
4. Combine the peppers, onions, and celery in a bowl.
5. Add the mayonnaise mixture and stir well.
6. Stir in the eggs and potatoes.
7. Let chill for 30-60 minutes.
8. Serve a generous 1/3 cup per serving.

Recipe tips:
- May sub Veganaise® for the mayo and a sweetener for the sugar.

Allergens:
Dairy, Eggs. (Check mayonnaise and Dijon mustard packages for allergens).

Nutrition Information:
Calculated using the NB2O system which is linked to the USDA database. Not lab tested so nutrition is not lab accurate. Calculated using 1 teaspoon garlic powder and standard Mayo (soybean based).

Calories: 144, Fat: 8g, Sat. Fat: 2g, Trans Fat: 0g, Cholesterol: 69mg, Carbohydrates: 16g, Fiber: 1g, Sugar: 4g, Sodium: 175mg, Protein: 3g, Calcium: 16mg, Phosphorus: 57mg, Potassium: 214mg

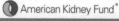 American Kidney Fund®

CKD Culinary Consulting

Recipe: sunshine salad

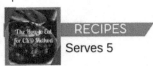

Serves 5

Sunshine Salad

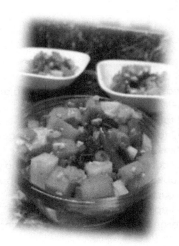

Ingredients:
1 large navel orange
1 tablespoon olive oil
1 teaspoon garlic, minced (1 clove)
1/16 teaspoon kosher salt
1/4 teaspoon ground nutmeg
1/4 teaspoon ground mustard
1/4 teaspoon white pepper (or black)
1 cup carrots, sliced
1 cup parsnips, sliced
1 cup green beans, cut into 1-inch pieces
1/4 cup green onion, sliced (about 2 medium, bulb and green)
3 tablespoons no salt, dry roasted peanuts, chopped
3 tablespoons golden raisins
2 tablespoons fresh basil, chopped

Instructions:
1. From the orange, reserve 2 teaspoons of zest. From half the orange, reserve 1/2 cup of flesh, chopped. From the other half of the orange, place 2 tablespoons of juice into a sealable jar or container.
   a. When juicing the orange, you do not need to strain out the pulp.
2. To the jar, add oil, garlic, salt, nutmeg, mustard, and white pepper. Shake vigorously and set aside.
3. Fill a large pot with water and bring to a boil. As that is heating, prepare your remaining ingredients.
4. When water is boiling, add the carrots, parsnips, and green beans. Stir to distribute, bring back to a boil and cook for 2 minutes.
   a. Beans should remain vibrant green and vegetables should still be crisp.
5. Drain the vegetables and immediately begin running cold water over top for 1 minute or they are cool.
6. Place all vegetables in a bowl, add the green onions, peanuts, raisins, basil, and the reserved orange zest and the flesh. Toss well.
7. Give the jar another good shake to combine the dressing then pour over the mix. Toss well and serve a generous 1/2 cup per person.

Recipe tips:
- May sub another nut for the peanuts.
- Add your favorite protein for a light meal.

Allergens: Peanut, Citrus.

Nutrition Information:
Calculated using the NB2O system which is linked to the USDA database. Not lab tested so nutrition is not lab accurate.

Calories: 126, Fat: 6g, Sat. Fat: 1g, Trans Fat: 0g, Cholesterol: 0mg, Carbohydrates: 18g, Fiber: 4g, Sugar: 9g, Sodium: 71mg, Protein: 3g, Calcium: 49mg, Phosphorus: 72mg, Potassium: 394mg

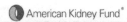

Recipe: mojito fruit salad

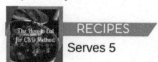

Serves 5

Mojito Fruit Salad

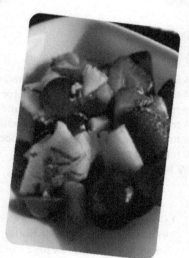

Ingredients:
1 cup red grapes, cut in half
1 cup strawberries, sliced
1 cup apple (1 medium)
1 teaspoon lime zest
1 tablespoon lime juice
1-ounce coconut water (2 tablespoons)
2 tablespoons fresh chopped mint

Instructions:
1. Cut the grapes in half then slice the berries. Peel and cut apple to similar size of the grapes.
2. In a large bowl, toss the apples with the lime juice.
3. Add remaining ingredients to the bowl and toss.
4. If desired, chill for 30 minutes before serving.
5. Serve 1/2 cup per person.

Recipe tips:
- Look for small to go containers of coconut water.
- May sub soda or sparkling water for the coconut water.

Allergens:
Strawberry, Coconut, Mint.

Nutrition Information:
Calculated using the NB2O system which is linked to the USDA database. Not lab tested so nutrition is not lab accurate. Calculated using Swerve® and cashews.

Calories: 41, Fat: 0g, Sat. Fat: 0g, Trans Fat: 0g, Cholesterol: 0mg, Carbohydrates: 10g, Fiber: 1g, Sugar: 8g, Sodium: 7mg, Protein: 1g, Calcium: 13mg, Phosphorus: 15mg, Potassium: 136mg

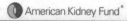

Recipe: no bake biscoff cookies

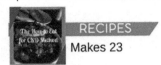 RECIPES

Makes 23

No Bake Biscoff® Cookies

Ingredients:
1 1/2 cup dry quick oats
4 tablespoons oat bran
4 tablespoons Swerve® granulated sweetener (or more sugar)
4 tablespoons granulated sugar (or more Swerve®)
6 tablespoons Biscoff® cookie butter
4 tablespoons unsalted butter, melted
2 tablespoons heavy cream (or coconut cream or nondairy)
2 tablespoons warm water
1/2 teaspoon vanilla

Instructions:
1. Combine the oats, bran, sweetener, and sugar together. Set aside.
2. In a bowl, mix the cookie butter, butter, cream, water, and vanilla until liquid is shiny and few lumps of butter left.
3. Stir the wet into the dry until well combined.
4. Scoop 1 tablespoon onto a baking sheet lined with parchment.
5. Freeze for 30 or chill for 60 minutes.
6. Keep cool. Cookies will soften as they remain at room temperature.
7. 1 serving = 1 cookie

Recipe tips:
- You could sub a nut butter for the cookie butter.
- You could add 3 tablespoons unsweetened cocoa powder to the dry mix.

Allergens:
Dairy. Wheat, Soy in Biscoff®.

Nutrition Information:
Calculated using the NB2O system which is linked to the USDA database. Not lab tested so nutrition is not lab accurate. Calculated using Swerve®, sugar, and heavy cream.

Calories: 75, Fat: 4g, Sat. Fat: 2g, Trans Fat: 0g, Cholesterol: 7mg, Carbohydrates: 9g, Fiber: 1g, Sugar: 4g, Sodium: 9mg, Protein: 1g, Calcium: 6mg, Phosphorus: 37mg, Potassium: 30mg

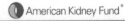

Recipe: banana cream dessert

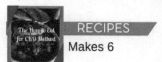

RECIPES

Makes 6

Banana Cream Dessert

Ingredients:
3-ounce box Jell-O® cook and serve banana cream flavored pudding
1/3 cup heavy cream
9 ounces water
6 tablespoons whipped topping
1 medium banana, cut into 18 slices
6 pack mini graham cracker crusts
12 teaspoons caramel sauce

Instructions:
1. Prepare pudding as directed on the box with the heavy cream and water.
2. Let pudding cool for 20 minutes.
3. As that is cooling, slice the banana into 18 pieces and place 2 slices into the bottom of each crust.
   a. *Reserve the remaining 6 for the top. Spritz with lemon juice to keep from browning and keep in the fridge.
4. When cooled for 20 minutes, divide the mixture between the 6 crusts.
5. If desired, let chill in the fridge for 10 minutes. If you prefer them warm, skip this step.
6. On each, place 1 tablespoon of whipped topping, 1 slice of banana, and drizzle 2 teaspoons of caramel over top.
7. Serve one mini pie per person.

Recipe tips:
• May sub sugar free and/or gluten free products.
• May omit the caramel.

Allergens:
Wheat/Gluten, Dairy. Check pudding, whipped topping, and caramel sauce for allergens.

Nutrition Information:
Calculated using the NB2O system which is linked to the USDA database. Not lab tested so nutrition is not lab accurate.

Calories: 265, Fat: 11g, Sat. Fat: 7g, Trans Fat: 0g, Cholesterol: 18mg, Carbohydrates: 41g, Fiber: 1g, Sugar: 26g, Sodium: 266mg, Protein: 2g, Calcium: 29mg, Phosphorus: 42mg, Potassium: 103mg

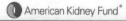

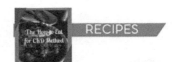 RECIPES

Gluten Free Recipes

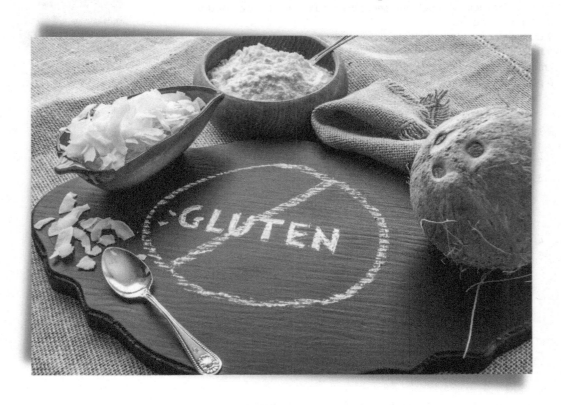

Sloppy Joe's

Fruit & Nut Broccoli Slaw

Gluten Free & Lower Carb Drop Biscuits

Chocolate Chip Sour Cream Coffee Cake

Recipe: gf sloppy joes

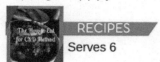

RECIPES
Serves 6

Sloppy Joe's

Ingredients:

2 tablespoons unsalted butter
1 pound ground beef or a 12-ounce bag of Quorn® meatless grounds
1/4 teaspoon ground star anise
1/2 teaspoon cinnamon
1 garlic clove, minced (about 1 teaspoon)
1/4 cup red onion, small dice
3 tablespoons no salt added tomato paste mixed with water to equal 1/2 cup
2 teaspoons Mrs. Dash® chicken griller blend
1 tablespoon gluten free Worcestershire sauce
2 tablespoons apple cider vinegar
2 tablespoons Swerve® brown sweetener or brown sugar
1/2 teaspoon ground coriander
1/2 teaspoon ground allspice
1/4 teaspoon kosher salt
1/2 teaspoon Embassa® chipotle adobo sauce
Up to 1 tablespoon arrowroot powder/starch/flour (if needed for thickening)
6 Gluten free buns

Instructions:

1. Place the butter into the InstaPot® and press sauté. Add the beef and cook halfway, pink should remain.
   a. *If you do not have an InstaPot® or pressure cooker, see tips below.
2. Place all remaining ingredients into the pot, except for arrowroot, and stir well.
   a. please note that you will be using the adobo sauce only, not the peppers.
3. Cook on high pressure for 20 minutes. Release pressure and stir well to fully combine all ingredients.
4. If liquid remains, mix enough arrowroot with 1 tablespoon of water, and stir it into the pot until thickened.
   a. If half cup liquid remains, use 1/2 tablespoon, if 1 cup liquid remains, use 1 tablespoon, etc.
   b. Arrowroot is used to thicken acidic ingredients. Cornstarch will not work as well.
5. Serve 1 ounce of meat per bun. 1 sandwich per serving.
   a. Suggested: serve with 1/4 cup dried cranberries drizzled with 1/2 teaspoon of honey or a mandarin orange cup.

Recipe tips:

- If you do not have an InstaPot®, you can use a large pan. Follow instructions above but cover and let simmer for 20-30 minutes, Stir occasionally. Then thicken if needed.
- *Arrowroot can be found in most grocery stores, possibly in the health foods isles or gluten free sections. It is called flour, powder, or starch.

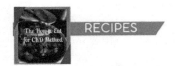 RECIPES

Sloppy Joe's

Allergens:
Dairy, tomato. Check Worcestershire for allergens. Mushroom, egg in Quorn®.

Nutrition Information:
Calculated using the NB2O system which is linked to the USDA database. Not lab tested so nutrition is not lab accurate. Calculated using 80% ground beef, Katz® buns, Embassa® (chipotles in) adobo sauce, sweetener and arrowroot.

Beef: Calories: 447, Fat: 27g, Sat. Fat: 12g, Trans Fat: 1g, Cholesterol: 134mg, Carbohydrates: 36g, Fiber: 1g, Sugar: 4g, Sodium: 367mg, Protein: 18g, Calcium: 51mg, Phosphorus: 152mg, Potassium: 403mg

Quorn®: Calories: 306, Fat: 13g, Sat. Fat: 6g, Trans Fat: 0g, Cholesterol: 80mg, Carbohydrates: 41g, Fiber: 5g, Sugar: 4g, Sodium: 342mg, Protein: 12g, Calcium: 134mg, Phosphorus: 163mg, Potassium: 242mg

If using the meatless crumbles suggested, you may be able to have two!
Serve with a side of fruit or vegetables, or check out my potato salad or vegan macaroni salad.

Recipe created for American Kidney Fund's Kidney Kitchen®, and contributed by Linda Blaylock of CKD Culinary Consulting, ©2019 all rights reserved.

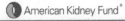 American Kidney Fund®

Recipe: fruit n nut broccoli slaw

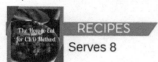

Serves 8

Fruit & Nut Broccoli Slaw

Ingredients:

12 ounces broccoli slaw

4 tablespoons (42g or 1 1/2oz) dried cherries

1/2 teaspoon lime zest

3 tablespoons (35g or 1 1/4oz) no salt dry roasted peanuts, halved, or crushed (or cashews)

4 tablespoons fresh lime juice

6 tablespoons peanut oil (or olive oil)

2 teaspoons dried tarragon

2 teaspoons dried oregano

2 teaspoons Swerve® powdered (or superfine caster sugar)

Instructions:

1. If desired, chop the slaw mix up to make it easier to eat.
2. Combine slaw mix, cherries, zest, and nuts in a large bowl.
3. In a sealable jar or container, add lime juice, oil, tarragon, oregano, and sugar.
   a. if using regular granulated sugar, it will take longer to dissolve, therefore, superfine is used. (Do not use powdered sugar)
4. Shake well until combined and pour over slaw mix.
5. Toss well and serve 1/2 cup per person.

Recipe tips:

- Add in pork or tempeh bacon for more flavor or a light meal.

Allergens:

Peanuts, if using.

Nutrition Information:

Calculated using the NB2O system which is linked to the USDA database. Not lab tested so nutrition is not lab accurate. Calculated using Swerve®, peanut oil, and peanuts.

Calories: 148, Fat: 12g, Sat. Fat: 2g, Trans Fat: 0g, Cholesterol: 0mg, Carbohydrates: 9g, Fiber: 2g, Sugar: 5g, Sodium: 14mg, Protein: 2g, Calcium: 31mg, Phosphorus: 50mg, Potassium: 200mg

Recipe created for American Kidney Fund's Kidney Kitchen®, and contributed by Linda Blaylock of CKD Culinary Consulting, ©2019 all rights reserved.

American Kidney Fund®

CKD Culinary Consulting

Recipe: gluten free, lower carb drop biscuits

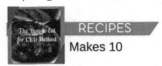

Makes 10

Gluten Free, Lower Carb Drop Biscuits

Ingredients:

2 ounces half and half (or nondairy)

1 tablespoon vinegar

1 ounce water

1/8 teaspoon coarse salt

1/2 cup (70g or 1 1/2oz) almond flour

1/4 cup (30g or 1oz) gluten free oat bran

1/4 cup (45g or 1 1/2oz) Bob's Red Mill® gluten free 1 to 1 flour (with xanthan)

1/4 teaspoon baking soda

1 teaspoon Swerve® powdered or superfine/baker's/caster sugar

3 tablespoons unsalted butter, melted (or vegan butter)

1/2 cup (58g) shredded cheddar cheese (or vegan shreds)

1 tablespoon unsalted butter, for brushing, melted (or vegan butter)

1/8 teaspoon garlic powder

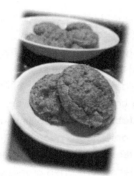

Recipe tips:

If desired, add 1/8 teaspoon garlic powder to the batter also.

Instructions:

1. Preheat the oven to 450° F / 232° C, and line a baking sheet with parchment.
2. Combine the half and half, vinegar, water, and salt. Set aside.
   a. If desired, use 3 ounces of buttermilk instead.
3. Mix the almond flour, oat bran, gluten free flour, baking soda, and sweetener, together.
4. Melt the 3 tablespoons of butter.
5. Pour the half and half mixture into the dry ingredients along with the melted butter, the cheese, and mix well.
6. Scoop 1 ounce (2T) sized biscuits onto the sheet. Let Rest 10 minutes.
7. Bake, upper rack, 12–15 minutes, or bottom edges are browned.
8. While that is baking, melt the tablespoon of butter and stir in the garlic powder. When biscuits come out of the oven, brush with the butter.
9. Let cool slightly on baking sheet. Best eaten when warm and/or same day.

Allergens:

Almond. Dairy, if using.

Nutrition Information:

Calculated using the NB20 system which is linked to the USDA database. Not lab tested so nutrition is not lab accurate. Calculated using Swerve®, dairy, and cheese.

Calories: 137, Fat: 11g, Sat. Fat: 5g, Trans Fat: 0g, Cholesterol: 20mg, Carbohydrates: 7g, Fiber: 1g, Sugar: 1g, Sodium: 120mg, Protein: 4g, Calcium: 71mg, Phosphorus: 98mg, Potassium: 86mg

Recipe created for American Kidney Fund's Kidney Kitchen®, and contributed by Linda Blaylock of CKD Culinary Consulting, ©2019 all rights reserved.

 American Kidney Fund®

recipesRecipe: gf choc chip sour cream coffee cake

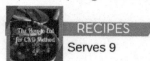

Serves 9

Gluten Free Chocolate Chip Sour Cream Coffee Cake

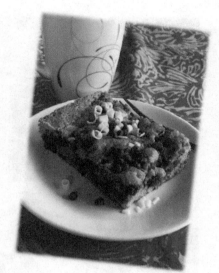

Ingredients:

BATTER

4 tablespoons unsalted butter, softened
1/4 (67g) cup brown sugar
1/4 cup (57g) granulated sugar
2 large eggs
1 cup (130g) Bob's Red Mill® gluten free 1 to 1 baking flour
1/2 teaspoon gluten free baking powder
1/2 teaspoon baking soda
1/8 teaspoon sea (kosher) salt
1/2 cup sour cream
1/2 teaspoon vanilla

FILLING

1/4 cup (67g) brown sugar
1/2 teaspoon ground cinnamon
3 ounces semi-sweet mini chocolate chips (enjoy life® suggested)

Instructions:

1. Preheat oven to 350° F / 177° C.
2. Combine butter, brown sugar, and sugar well.
3. Add only one egg and mix until incorporated.
4. Sift the flour, baking powder, baking soda, and salt together. Add half into the batter mix and beat until well mixed.
5. Add the sour cream and vanilla. Mix well.
6. Add the remaining flour and mix until well combined.
7. Add the second egg and beat well.
8. Grease an 8 x 8 pan or line with parchment, and pour 60% of the batter in.
9. Combine the brown sugar, cinnamon, and chocolate chips and sprinkle 60% over top of the batter.
10. Dot the remaining batter on top, and with a knife or spatula, swirl it in.
11. Top with the remaining filling mix.
12. Bake on middle rack for 30 minutes or toothpick comes clean from the middle and the sides have started to pull away from the pan. Turn oven off and leave in the oven for 10 minutes.
13. Remove and let cool. Cut into 9 pieces.

 RECIPES

Holiday Recipes

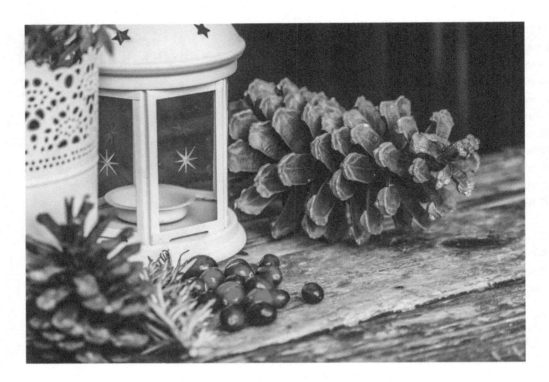

Green Bean Casserole

Wild Rice Stuffing

Hash Brown Casserole

Warm Spiced Root Veggies

Cranberry Bars

Cream Cheese Pumpkin Muffins

Recipe: green bean casserole

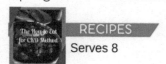

Serves 8

Green Bean Casserole

Ingredients:

1 1/2 tablespoons unsalted butter or vegan unsalted butter

1 1/2 tablespoons gluten free flour (or regular flour)

1 1/4 cups no salt added chicken broth or water

4 ounces heavy cream (or nondairy milk)

1/8 teaspoon white pepper or black

1/8 teaspoon ground nutmeg

1/4 teaspoon ground allspice

1/4 teaspoon ground dry mustard

2 teaspoons lower sodium Worcestershire sauce

4 ounces shredded sharp cheddar cheese (or vegan cheese shreds)

4 strips of reduced sodium bacon, diced (or tempeh bacon)

1/4 cup onion, diced

1 teaspoon sugar

3 cans no salt added cut green beans, (about 4 1/2 cups), drained

2.5-ounces gluten free crispy fried onions

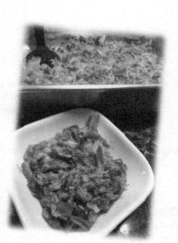

Instructions:

1. Preheat the oven to 350° F / 177° C.
2. To make the sauce: melt the butter in a saucepan over medium heat.
3. Whisk in the flour and cook 1-2 minutes, or until it is sand-like consistency.
4. Whisk in the broth and heavy cream. Continue whisking until flour has dissolved then add the pepper, nutmeg, salt, allspice, ground mustard, and Worcestershire.
5. *If you are using tempeh bacon, omit salt from the sauce.
6. Bring to a boil and cook 1-2 minutes or it begins to thicken. Turn off the heat and whisk in the cheddar until fully melted and combined. The sauce should still be pourable yet thick enough to see some trails from the whisk.
7. *If using vegan cheese, add 2 tablespoons of Nutritional Yeast to the sauce with the cheese shreds.
8. In a large pan add diced bacon, onion, and sugar. Turn heat to medium. Cook until the bacon is crisp around the edges and the fat is bubbling.
9. Add the green beans and toss until beans are warm and coated with the fat, 1-2 minutes.
10. Place bean and bacon mix into a casserole dish or 9 x 13 pan and pour sauce over top.
11. Crumble the fried onions in your hand as you sprinkle them over top.
12. Bake for 30 minutes or fried onions are golden, and sauce is bubbling.
13. *If desired, mix in your favorite protein for a full meal.
14. Let rest 10 minutes or more before serving so sauce has a chance to thicken.

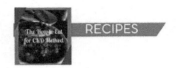

Green Bean Casserole

Recipe tips:
- The fried onions really make this dish, it is worth it to seek them out, try Whole Foods. You could sub gluten free panko breadcrumbs or lightly salted crushed potato chips, gluten free crackers, or gluten free pretzels for the fried onions.

Allergens:
Dairy, Cheese. Check broth, Worcestershire, and fried onions (if using) for allergens.

Nutrition Information:
Calculated using the NB2O system which is linked to the USDA database. Not lab tested so nutrition is not lab accurate. Calculated using Bob's Red Mill® 1 to 1 gluten free flour and Full Circle Market® gluten free fried onions, and dairy products.

Calories: 235, Fat: 18g, Sat. Fat: 9g, Trans Fat: 0g, Cholesterol: 44mg, Carbohydrates: 13g, Fiber: 2g, Sugar: 2g, Sodium: 199mg, Protein: 8g, Calcium: 150mg, Phosphorus: 134mg, Potassium: 204mg

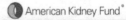

recipesRecipe: wild rice stuffing

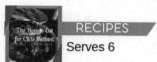

Serves 6

Wild Rice Stuffing

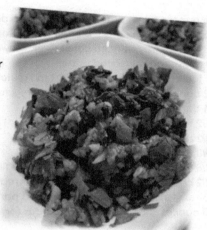

Ingredients:

16-ounces cooked wild rice

5-ounces of riced cauliflower risotto or medley mix, cooked

2-ounces no salt dry roasted peanuts, chopped (or another nut)

4-ounces lower sodium bacon, diced and cooked to near crisp (or tempeh bacon)

Grease from the cooked bacon, about 3 tablespoons (use oil to equal 3T if need)

1/2 cup (4 oz) no salt added canned mushrooms, drained

1 teaspoon ground sage

1 teaspoon dried marjoram

3/4 teaspoon dried tarragon

1/2 teaspoon dried thyme

1/4 teaspoon garlic powder

1/4 teaspoon poultry seasoning

1/8 teaspoon kosher salt

1/4 cup fresh parsley, chopped

Instructions:

1. Preheat the oven to 375° F / 191° C.
2. Mix everything together, except the parsley.
   a. If using tempeh bacon, or higher sodium bacon, or salted nuts, omit the kosher salt.
   b. If using tempeh bacon, add 4 tablespoons of oil to the stuffing mixture to sub for the bacon grease.
   c. If using frozen or fresh mushrooms, cook and measure 4-ounces after cooking.
3. Place in a greased casserole dish or an 8x8 pan and bake for 30 minutes.
4. Garnish with fresh parsley. Serve 1/2 cup per person.

Recipe tips:

- If not concerned with carbs, you may sub 1/2 cup of brown rice for the cauliflower.
- Add a little extra butter or oil when reheating.

Allergens:

Nuts, if using.

Nutrition Information:

Calculated using the NB2O system which is linked to the USDA database. Not lab tested so nutrition is not lab accurate. Calculated using peanuts, bacon, bacon grease.

Calories: 248, Fat: 19g, Sat. Fat: 3g, Trans Fat: 0g, Cholesterol: 6mg, Carbohydrates: 14g, Fiber: 2g, Sugar: 2g, Sodium: 190mg, Protein: 8g, Calcium: 24mg, Phosphorus: 128mg, Potassium: 299mg

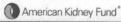

Recipe: hashbrown casserole

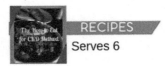

Serves 6

Hashbrown Casserole

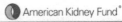

Ingredients:

6 ounces sweet potatoes, peeled and diced
6 ounces no salt added canned potatoes
8 ounces frozen riced cauliflower, thawed (or broccoli)
1 tablespoon unsalted butter
1 tablespoon Bob's Red Mill® 1 to 1 gluten free flour (or regular flour)
2 ounces heavy cream (or nondairy sour cream)
4 ounces water
1/2 teaspoon garlic powder
1/2 teaspoon onion powder
1/8 teaspoon white pepper (or black)
1/8 teaspoon cayenne (or red pepper flakes)
1/2 cup sour cream (or vegan sour cream)
3 tablespoons lower sodium grated parmesan (or vegan parmesan)
3 ounces shredded sharp cheddar (or vegan shreds)

Instructions:

1. Preheat the oven to 350° F / 177° C.
2. Toss the potatoes and cauliflower together. Set aside.
3. In a large saucepan over medium heat, melt the butter. When melted, whisk in the flour, and cook until sand-like consistency. 1-2 minutes.
4. Pour in the cream, water, and all seasonings.
5. Whisk and cook until the mixture begins to thicken. 1-3 minutes, depending on your pan size and heat level.
6. Remove from heat and whisk in the sour cream, parmesan, and 1 ounce of the cheddar cheese.
7. Add the vegetables and mix well.
8. Place into a greased casserole dish or an 8x8 baking pan. Top with the remaining cheddar.
9. Cover with foil and bake for 30 minutes.
10. Remove foil and bake another 15-25 minutes or hot and bubbly and vegetables are tender crisp.
11. Let stand 10-15 minutes for the sauce to settle and thicken.
12. Serve a generous 1/2 cup per person.

Recipe tips:

- If not concerned with carbs, you may increase both potatoes by 4 ounces.

Allergens:

Cheese, Dairy.

Nutrition Information:

Calculated using the NB2O system which is linked to the USDA database. Not lab tested so nutrition is not lab accurate. Calculated using cauliflower, gluten free flour, dairy, white pepper, and cayenne.

Calories: 216, Fat: 15g, Sat. Fat: 9g, Trans Fat: 0g, Cholesterol: 45mg, Carbohydrates: 15g, Fiber: 3g, Sugar: 3g, Sodium: 169mg, Protein: 7g, Calcium: 174mg, Phosphorus: 162mg, Potassium: 341mg

Recipe: warm spiced root veggies

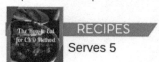

RECIPES
Serves 5

Warm Spiced Root Veggies

Ingredients:

8 ounces sweet potatoes, diced
8 ounces carrots, diced
1 tablespoon oil
1 teaspoon ground ginger
1/2 teaspoon allspice
1/4 plus 1/8 teaspoon chili seasoning mix
1/8 teaspoon kosher salt
1 cup (5 ounces) sweet-tangy apple, diced
1/2 teaspoon lemon juice
1/2 teaspoon fennel seeds (or anise seed), slightly crushed
1 tablespoon oil
1 tablespoon apple cider vinegar
2 tablespoons fresh parsley, chopped

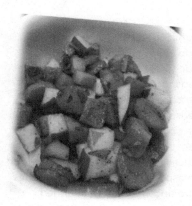

Instructions:

1. Preheat the oven to 425° F / 218° C.
2. Toss the sweet potatoes and carrots with the oil, ginger, allspice, chili seasoning, and salt.
   a. Make sure the potatoes, carrots, and apples are cut to about the same size.
3. Place on a foil lined baking sheet. Roast on the top rack for 20-30 minutes or tender.
4. While that is roasting, dice the apple and toss with lemon juice to prevent browning.
5. In a small skillet over medium heat, add the fennel seeds. Toast for 1-2 minutes, tossing constantly, until fragrant. Set aside.
6. Whisk the oil and vinegar together until well combined. Add the fennel seeds, whisk, and let stand.
7. When vegetables are done, add the apples and parsley and toss well.
8. Whisk the dressing again to recombine then drizzle it over top of the vegetables and toss to combine.
9. Serve 1/2 cup per person.

Recipe tips:
- If need, make sure your chili seasoning is gluten free.
- This taste amazing with fried bacon or diced pork chops added in.

Allergens:
Check chili powder seasoning mix for allergens.

Nutrition Information:
Calculated using the NB2O system which is linked to the USDA database. Not lab tested so nutrition is not lab accurate. Calculated using olive oil and Mrs. Dash® chili seasoning.

Calories: 125, Fat: 6g, Sat. Fat: 1g, Trans Fat: 0g, Cholesterol: 0mg, Carbohydrates: 18g, Fiber: 4g, Sugar: 7g, Sodium: 82mg, Protein: 7g, Calcium: 37mg, Phosphorus: 43mg, Potassium: 352mg

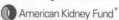

recipesRecipe: gf lc cranberry bars

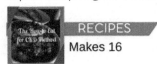

Makes 16

Cranberry Bars (GF, LC)

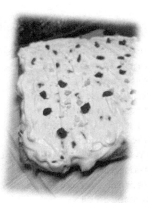

Ingredients:

BASE
1/2 cup (58g) almond flour
1/4 cup (20g) gluten free oat bran
1/4 cup (30g) pecans, chopped
1/2 teaspoon baking powder
1/2 teaspoon ground ginger
1/4 teaspoon ground nutmeg
1/4 teaspoon ground allspice
1/8 teaspoon coarse salt
2 ounces (60g) Lily's® no sugar added white chocolate chips
2 tablespoons (25g) dried cranberries
1/4 cup unsalted butter, softened
4 tablespoons (40g) Swerve® granular
4 tablespoons (32g) Allulose sweetener (or more Swerve®)
2 large eggs
3/4 teaspoon orange extract
1/2 teaspoon vanilla extract
1/8 teaspoon almond extract
1/2 teaspoon orange zest

TOPPING
2 ounces cream cheese, room temperature
4 ounces mascarpone cheese (or more cream cheese)
2 ounces heavy cream
4 tablespoons (40g) Swerve® powdered
3/4 teaspoon orange extract
1/2 teaspoon vanilla extract
1/2 teaspoon orange zest
2 tablespoons (25g) dried cranberries
1 1/2 ounces (45g) Lily's® no sugar added white chocolate chips

Instructions:

1. Preheat oven to 350° F / 177° C. Line an 9x9 pan with parchment.
2. In a food processor, process the almond flour, oat bran, pecans, baking powder, ginger, nutmeg, allspice, salt, chocolate chips, and cranberries, until pecans, chocolate and cranberries are in small bits.
3. Add the butter, sweeteners, eggs, extracts, and zest. Process until well combined.
4. Pour into the pan, spread evenly, and bake 25-30 or edges just start to turn brown. Remove and let cool completely.
5. As that is cooling, make the topping: beat the cream cheese, mascarpone, heavy cream, sweetener, extracts, and zest together until smooth, 1-2 minutes on medium speed.
6. Stir in the cranberries and chocolate. If desired, remove 1 tablespoon of each and chop for garnish.
   a. If using all cream cheese and the mixture is too thick, add 1 tablespoons of water at a time until desired consistency. Should be thick but spreadable.
7. Spread evenly over the fully cooled bars.
   a. If desired, chill before serving.
8. Cut into 16 bars.

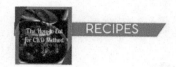

Cranberry Bars

Recipe tips:
- May use cashews instead of pecans, may use cherries instead of cranberries. (Will raise carbs and other nutrition values).

Allergens:
Nuts. Chocolate, Cheese, Citrus.

Nutrition Information:
Calculated using the NB2O system which is linked to the USDA database. Not lab tested so nutrition is not lab accurate. Calculated using Allulose and mascarpone.

Half of the sweetener carbs are counted in recipe as our body digests half of them.

Calories: 169, Fat: 15g, Sat. Fat: 7g, Trans Fat: 0g, Cholesterol: 50mg, Carbohydrates: 9g, Fiber: 2g, Sugar: 3g, Sodium: 79mg, Protein: 3g, Calcium: 55mg, Phosphorus: 76mg, Potassium: 94mg

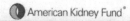

American Kidney Fund®

CKD Culinary Consulting

Recipe: cream cheese pumpkin muffins

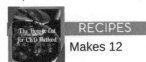

Makes 12

Cream Cheese Pumpkin Muffins (GF, LC)

Ingredients:

BATTER:

12 tablespoons (3.25 oz) pecan halves, chopped small or ground (or another nut)

2-ounces whipped cream cheese

2-ounces crème fraîche

1/2 cup (4.75 oz) pumpkin puree

4 tablespoons (1.85 oz) Swerve® brown sweetener

1 large egg

1 teaspoon vanilla

1 teaspoon pumpkin pie spice

1/4 teaspoon allspice

1/8 teaspoon coarse salt

2 tablespoons chickpea flour

FROSTING:

4-ounces whipped cream cheese

2 tablespoons unsalted butter, softened

1 ounce (2T) crème fraîche

6 tablespoons Swerve® powdered sweetener

1 tablespoon pumpkin puree

1/4 teaspoon vanilla

1/8 teaspoon nutmeg

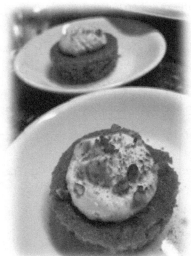

Instructions:

1. Preheat the oven to 350º F / 177º C.
2. Line a muffin tin with cupcake liners and place 1 tablespoon of chopped or ground pecans at the bottom of each.
3. In a large bowl, beat the cream cheese, crème fraîche, pumpkin puree, sweetener, egg, vanilla, pie spice, allspice, and salt together until well combined. Add the flour and mix until it just comes together.
4. Scoop 1 ounce (2 T) into each muffin liner.
5. Bake 20-25 minutes, middle rack, until tops look dry and no batter sticks to your finger when touched.
6. Remove and let cool just until they have cooled enough to handle, then place into the fridge for at least 45 minutes to fully set.
7. As that is cooling, Beat the frosting ingredients together until well combined. Chill until ready to use.
8. Top each muffin with frosting.
   a. Optional: sprinkle ground nuts and cinnamon on top

CKD Culinary Consulting

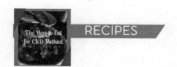

RECIPES

Cream Cheese Pumpkin Muffins

Recipe tips:
- If desired, add 1/4 cup diced dried cranberries or cherries to the batter. You may reduce the amount of the nuts used but do not omit!

Allergens:
Nut, Dairy, Cheese, Egg.

Nutrition Information:
Calculated using the NB2O system which is linked to the USDA database. Not lab tested so nutrition is not lab accurate. Calculated using pecans and full fat dairy.
Additional nuts and cinnamon not included.

Half of the sweetener carbs are counted in recipe as our body digests half of them.

Calories: 318, Fat: 15g, Sat. Fat: 6g, Trans Fat: 0g, Cholesterol: 42mg, Carbohydrates: 7g, Fiber: 1g, Sugar: 1g, Sodium: 92mg, Protein: 3g, Calcium: 31mg, Phosphorus: 57mg, Potassium: 98mg

Recipe created for American Kidney Fund's Kidney Kitchen®, and contributed by Linda Blaylock of CKD Culinary Consulting, ©2021 all rights reserved.

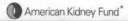

American Kidney Fund®

CKD Culinary Consulting

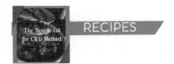 RECIPES

Lower Carb Recipes

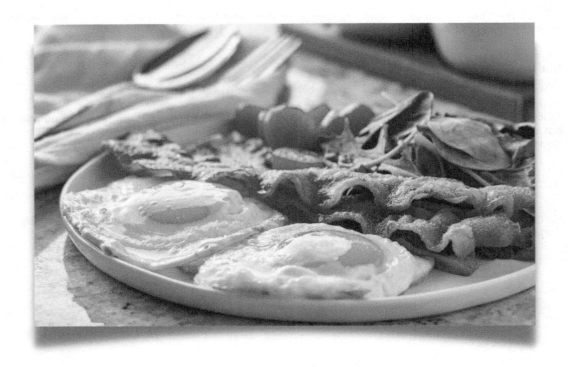

Southwest Breakfast Tacos

Polenta & Egg Breakfast Cups

Hush Puppies

Egg Roll Bowl

Spiced Meringue Cookies

Recipe: lc southwest breakfast tacos

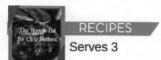

Serves 3

Southwest Breakfast Tacos

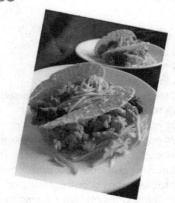

Ingredients:
6 taco shells (La Tiara® recommended)
3 large eggs (or 9T JUST egg sub)
1 3/4 teaspoons Mrs. Dash® taco seasoning
1/8 teaspoon sea salt (omit if using shells with sodium)
4 tablespoons red bell pepper, diced
4 tablespoons tomatoes, diced
4 tablespoons corn kernels (preferably fresh but can use no salt added canned)
1 tablespoon unsalted butter
6 tablespoons shredded cheddar cheese (2 ounces)
6 tablespoons of cilantro (optional)

Instructions:
1. Place the shells on the rack in the oven and turn the oven to warm or 170° F / 77° C. Remove shells from the oven when oven reaches temperature.
2. Mix the eggs and seasonings until frothy. Stir in peppers, tomatoes, and corn.
3. Melt the butter in a large pan over medium-low heat and add the eggs.
4. Cook, stirring often, until eggs are set but still appear moist and creamy. 2–3 minutes.
5. Remove from heat, stir a few more times, then set aside.
6. Place 3 tablespoons of eggs into each shell. Top each with 1 tablespoon of cheese.
7. Top each with 1 tablespoon of cilantro.
8. Serve 2 tacos per person.

Recipe tips:
- La Tiara® shells are recommended as they are very thin and contain no sodium. Thicker shells would overpower the flavors and textures of the filling.
- If desired, serve each person 1/4 cup of either: fresh cherries, strawberries, apples, raspberries, nectarines, or peaches, or a combination thereof.

Allergens:
Corn, Eggs, Tomato, Cheese. Yeast in Mrs. Dash® seasoning.

Nutrition Information:
Calculated using the NB2O system which is linked to the USDA database. Not lab tested so nutrition is not lab accurate. Calculated using la tiara® shells, Mrs. Dash® seasoning, canned corn, and eggs. Does not include cilantro.

Calories: 282, Fat: 19g, Sat. Fat: 10g, Trans Fat: 2g, Cholesterol: 216mg, Carbohydrates: 13g, Fiber: 1g, Sugar: 2g, Sodium: 352mg, Protein: 12g, Calcium: 189mg, Phosphorus: 247mg, Potassium: 216mg

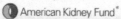

Recipe: lc polenta n egg breakfast cups

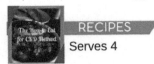

RECIPES

Serves 4

Polenta & Egg Breakfast Cups

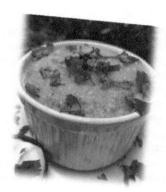

Ingredients:
6 ounces polenta log/chub
4 teaspoons unsalted butter
4 large eggs
2 teaspoons Mrs. Dash® taco seasoning
1/8 teaspoon sea (kosher) salt
1/4 cup small diced red pepper
1/4 cup small diced roma tomatoes
1/4 cup thin sliced green onions (about 2 medium)
2 ounces shredded cheddar cheese, divided
2 tablespoons cilantro, chopped
2 tablespoons Mexican crema or sour cream

Instructions:

1. Preheat the oven to 500° F / 260° C.
2. Cut polenta into four, 1 1/2-ounce servings (about 1/2-inch-thick slices). Crumble into greased ramekin cups.
3. Top each with 1 teaspoon of butter and broil 6-9 minutes or hot and bubbling.
4. Whisk together the eggs, taco seasoning, salt, red pepper, and onions.
5. Remove ramekins from oven and reduce oven heat to 400° F / 204° C.
6. Sprinkle 1 tablespoon of cheese on top of the polenta in each ramekin.
7. Divide the egg mixture between the ramekins and bake 12-18 minutes or eggs are set (no wobbly middle) but still look moist.
8. Remove from oven and top each with 1 tablespoon of remaining cheese and let rest 2-3 minutes.
9. Top with 1/2 tablespoon each of cilantro and crema or sour cream.

Recipe tips:
- May sub parsley for cilantro.

Allergens:
Corn, Dairy, Cheese, Eggs, Tomatoes. Yeast in Mrs. Dash® seasoning.

Nutrition Information:
Calculated using the NB2O system which is linked to the USDA database. Not lab tested so nutrition is not lab accurate. Calculated using sour cream.

Calories: 216, Fat: 15g, Sat. Fat: 8g, Trans Fat: 0g, Cholesterol: 215mg, Carbohydrates: 9g, Fiber: 1g, Sugar: 1g, Sodium: 395mg, Protein: 11g, Calcium: 148mg, Phosphorus: 195mg, Potassium: 172mg

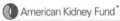

Recipe: lc hushpuppies

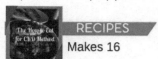

RECIPES

Makes 16

Hush Puppies

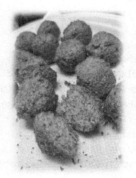

Ingredients:

2 tablespoons heavy cream

2 tablespoons water

2 teaspoon vinegar

3/4 cup (90g) almond flour

2 tablespoons (15g) cup oat bran

1/4 cup (32g) corn meal

1/4 teaspoon baking soda

1/2 teaspoon garlic powder

1/2 teaspoon onion powder

1/4 teaspoon coarse salt

1/4 teaspoon white pepper

1/8 teaspoon cayenne

2 teaspoons (5g) Swerve® powdered

1 egg, beaten

1 teaspoon cornbread extract

Instructions:

1. Begin heating 1-inch of oil to 325° to 350° F / 163° to 177° C, using a large pot, pan, or use a deep fryer.
2. Mix the heavy cream, water, and vinegar together. Set aside.
3. Whisk the almond flour, oat bran, cornmeal, baking soda, all seasonings, and the sweetener together.
4. Beat the egg and extract into the cream mixture, then add to the dry ingredients. Mix just until it comes together.
5. Scoop 1 tablespoon size balls into the pot and fry 1-2 minutes per side, or golden brown. Make sure to adjust your heat as needed.
6. Place on a paper towel lined pan to drain.
7. Serve with any sauce you wish.
8. 1 puppy = 1 serving. Best when warm, and same day.

Recipe tips:
- May replace the cornmeal with more almond flour.
- May use 2 ounces of buttermilk instead of the heavy cream, water, and vinegar mixture.
- Cornbread extract can be found online.

Allergens:
Nuts, Corn, Egg, Dairy.

Nutrition Information:
Calculated using the NB2O system which is linked to the USDA database. Not lab tested so nutrition is not lab accurate.

Calories: 56, Fat: 4g, Sat. Fat: 1g, Trans Fat: 0g, Cholesterol: 14mg, Carbohydrates: 4g, Fiber: 1g, Sugar: 1g, Sodium: 85mg, Protein: 2g, Calcium: 19mg, Phosphorus: 44mg, Potassium: 54mg

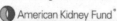

Recipe: lc egg roll bowl

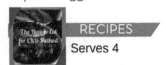

RECIPES

Serves 4

Egg Roll Bowl

Ingredients:

1 tablespoon sesame seeds
2 tablespoons sesame oil, divided
1 garlic clove, minced (1 teaspoon)
1 tablespoon fresh ginger, minced and divided
1/2-pound ground pork
1/2 cup red onion, sliced thin
1/2 cup carrots, shredded
3 cups (170g) shredded cabbage or coleslaw mix

2 teaspoons lower sodium soy sauce
1 tablespoon lower sodium Worcestershire sauce
1 1/2 teaspoons Coconut Secret® coconut aminos
1 teaspoon fish sauce
1 tablespoon Taco Bell® hot sauce
2 green onions, sliced thin (1/4 cup)
10-ounce bag riced cauliflower, cooked

Instructions:

1. In a small non-stick skillet over medium-low heat, add the sesame seeds and toss constantly for 1 minute, until seeds begin to turn golden. Do not use oil. Set aside.
2. In a large skillet over medium heat, add 1 tablespoon of the sesame oil. When hot, add garlic and half the ginger. Stir and cook for 30 seconds or fragrant.
3. Add the pork and cook 4-5 minutes or no longer pink.
4. Add the remaining sesame oil, the onions and carrots, and cook 3 minutes.
5. Add the soy sauce, Worcestershire, aminos, fish sauce, and hot sauce. Simmer 5 minutes.
6. Add 1/2 the cabbage and cook about 2 minutes, until cabbage is tender-crisp.
7. Remove from heat and stir in the green onions, cauliflower, remaining ginger, remaining cabbage, and the toasted sesame seeds.
8. Divide between four bowls and serve immediately.

Recipe tips:
- Use Ocean's Halo® fish free fish sauce.
- Use 12 oz of pork if protein, potassium, and phosphorus are less restrictive.
- May use 12 ounces of Quorn® meatless crumbles as a vegetarian option, or use tempeh, seitan, or canned jackfruit for a vegan option.

Allergens:
Sesame, Coconut (in aminos), Fish (in fish sauce). Check soy sauce, Worcestershire sauce, and hot sauce for allergens.

Nutrition Information:
Calculated using the NB2O system which is linked to the USDA database. Not lab tested so nutrition is not lab accurate. Calculated using cabbage.

Calories: 315, Fat: 22 g, Saturated Fat: 6 g, Trans Fat: 0 g, Cholesterol: 58 mg, Carbs: 12 g, Sugar: 6 g, Fiber: 4 g, Protein: 19 g, Sodium: 415 mg, Calcium: 70 mg, Phosphorus: 206 mg, Potassium: 587 mg.

Recipe: lc spiced meringue cookies

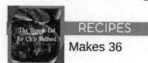

RECIPES

Makes 36

Spiced Meringue Cookies

Ingredients:
1/2 teaspoon ground cinnamon
1/2 teaspoon ground ginger
1/8 teaspoon allspice
1/8 teaspoon ground nutmeg
1 tablespoon caster / superfine / baker's sugar and 1 tablespoon of
Swerve® powdered sweetener (see tips for grams and reasons)
2 large egg whites, room temp
1/8 teaspoon cream of tartar or lemon juice
1/4 tsp vanilla extract
2 tablespoons chopped dried fruits and/or nuts (optional)

Instructions:
1. Preheat the oven to 250° F / 121° C.
2. Wet a paper towel with some vinegar or lemon juice and wipe out a metal or glass mixing bowl and the whisk of your mixer. (Egg whites will not whip if any fat is present. Vinegar helps remove any unseen fat there may be. They also do not like plastic).
   a. If eggs are not at room temperature, place them into a bowl of warm water for 5 minutes before using.
3. Place the egg whites and cream of tartar (or lemon juice) into the bowl. Whisk on medium until the whites are frothy. Begin adding 1 tbsp of sugar, waiting 3-5 seconds, then the next.
4. When sugar is added, increase speed to medium-high and beat 2-3 minutes or the whites are shiny and form stiff peaks.
   a. When lifting the whisk, the whites should stand up and not fall over.
   b. If you do not have caster sugar, run your granulated through a grinder until it is very fine. Powdered sugar is not acceptable.
   c. You will know the whites are nearly ready when there are thick trails from the whisk.
   d. If adding chopped nuts or fruits, gently fold in now.
5. Gently place into a piping bag, and pipe 1-inch sized mounds onto a parchment lined baking sheet, about 1 inch high.
6. Bake one hour without opening the door. Turn off oven and let them remain for at least thirty minutes or until oven is cold.
7. Best within the first day. They will start to accumulate moisture and become soft and chewy over time.

Recipe tips:
- Plastic holds fat and whites can struggle to whip in them. Therefore, glass, metal, or ceramic is best.
- These need the strength and structure that sugar provides. Not recommended to use all sweetener if using half and half, do 70 g of caster and 100g of sweetener (measured using Swerve®).

Allergens: Eggs.

Nutrition Information:
Calculated using the NB2O system which is linked to the USDA database. Not lab tested so nutrition is not lab accurate. Does not include chopped nuts or fruits. Per cookie:

Calories: 10, Fat: 0g, Sat. Fat: 0g, Trans Fat: 0g, Cholesterol: 0mg, Carbohydrates: 2g, Fiber: 0g, Sugar: 2g, Sodium: 3mg, Protein: 0g, Calcium: 0.54mg, Phosphorus: 0.36mg, Potassium: 5mg

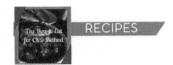 RECIPES

Vegan & Vegetarian Recipes

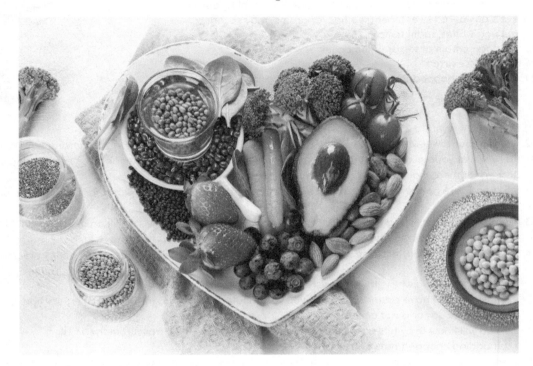

Vegan Tofu Tortilla Soup

Fiesta Veggie Bowl

Vegan Sweet Potatoes & Quinoa

Macaroni Salad

Mango Raspberry Yogurt Cup

Recipe: vegan tortilla soup

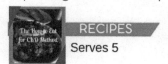

Serves 5

Vegan Tofu Tortilla Soup

Ingredients:

7 ounces firm tofu

2 tablespoons oil

1/2 cup red onion, chopped

1/4 cup jalapeno, diced. De-seed and de-vein, if desired

1 garlic clove, minced (1 teaspoon)

1 cup red bell pepper, chopped

1 cup canned hominy, drained, and rinsed well

1 tablespoon Mrs. Dash® taco seasoning

1 teaspoon ground cinnamon

1 teaspoon garlic powder

1 teaspoon ground cumin

1/2 teaspoon white pepper

1/8 teaspoon sea (kosher) salt

1/8 teaspoon ground allspice

1 teaspoon chipotle in adobo sauce (sauce only)

1 cup tomatoes, chopped

2 cups low sodium vegetable broth

1/2 cup water

10 ounces frozen riced cauliflower (may use 1 cup cooked rice)

1 cup no salt added canned corn, drained (may use frozen)

2 tablespoons lime juice

5 tablespoons nondairy sour cream like Kite Hill®

1/2 cup fresh cilantro, chopped

2 soft corn tortillas

Instructions:

1. Press the tofu between two plates and place something heavy on top to release extra liquid as you prep your ingredients. Drain, pat dry and cut into 1-inch cubes.
2. Heat oil in a large pot over medium heat and add onions. Cook 3-4 minutes or they begin to soften.
3. Add the tofu and cook 3-4 minutes or edges start to brown.
4. Add the jalapenos, garlic, bell pepper, and hominy. Cook 2-3 minutes or hominy is fragrant.
5. Add all the seasonings, adobo, and tomatoes. Cook for 2 minutes, stirring constantly.
6. Add the broth, water, and cauliflower. If using frozen corn, add now as well.
7. Bring to a boil, reduce heat and simmer, covered, for 10 minutes.
8. Turn off heat. If using canned corn, add now.
    a. If using precooked rice instead of cauliflower, add now.
9. Add lime juice and stir well.
10. Place cover back on and let stand 5 minutes.
11. Serve generous 1 1/2 cups each, with 1 tablespoon nondairy sour cream, 3/4 tablespoon cilantro, and tortilla triangles.

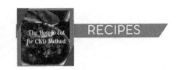

Vegan Tofu Tortilla Soup

Recipe tips:
- Omit tortillas to bring carbs to 23.
- Sub parsley, tarragon, dill, or a combination thereof, for cilantro.
- Serve with 1/4 cup per person of fresh strawberries, raspberries, or combination thereof.

Allergens:
Tomatoes, Corn, Soy. Yeast (in Mrs. Dash® seasoning). Check broth, adobo, nondairy sour cream, and tortillas for allergens.

Nutrition Information:
Calculated using the NB2O system which is linked to the USDA database. Not lab tested so nutrition is not lab accurate. Calculated using white hominy, Nasoya® tofu, and Forager® nondairy sour cream, cauliflower, and canned corn. Phosphorus for nondairy sour cream is estimated.

Calories: 220, Fat: 10g, Sat. Fat: 2g, Trans Fat: 0g, Cholesterol: 0mg, Carbohydrates: 28g, Fiber: 6g, Sugar: 6g, Sodium: 307mg, Protein: 8g, Calcium: 118mg, Phosphorus: 166mg, Potassium: 492mg

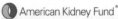

Recipe: fiesta veggie bowl

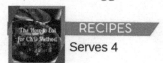

RECIPES
Serves 4

Fiesta Veggie Bowl

Ingredients:

1 1/2 cups (15 ounce can) no salt added black beans
4 tablespoons nondairy sour cream or regular sour cream
4 tablespoons taco sauce
1/8 teaspoon kosher salt
5 ounces shredded lettuce
1 cup bell pepper, diced
1 cup roma tomatoes, diced
1/4 cup jalapenos, seeds, pith removed, diced
1/4 cup fresh cilantro, chopped
1/4 cup green onions, sliced (about 2 full medium)
1/4 cup radishes, chopped
2 ounces vegan shredded cheddar cheese or regular shredded cheddar
1-ounce corn chips (like Frito's®), crushed

Instructions:

1. Drain and rinse the black beans. Set aside. If desired, you may warm them.
2. Mix the sour cream, taco sauce, and salt together.
3. In a large bowl, toss the beans, lettuce, bell pepper, tomato, jalapeno, cilantro, onion, radishes, and cheese together then add the sauce and mix well.
4. Serve 1 1/4 cups per person with 1 tablespoon of corn chips on top.
5. If desired, serve with 1/4 cup sliced strawberries.

Recipe tips:

- Reduce cheese to 1 ounce and/or omit corn chips to reduce sodium.

Allergens:

Dairy, Tomato, Cheese. Corn in corn chips. Check the taco sauce you are using, for allergens.

Nutrition Information:

Calculated using the NB2O system which is linked to the USDA database. Not lab tested so nutrition is not lab accurate. Calculated using Forager® nondairy sour cream, Old El Paso® taco sauce, Daiya® nondairy cheddar cheese. Phosphorus for nondairy sour cream is estimated.

Calories: 239, Fat: 10g, Sat. Fat: 5g, Trans Fat: 0g, Cholesterol: 22mg, Carbohydrates: 27g, Fiber: 9g, Sugar: 5g, Sodium: 334mg, Protein: 11g, Calcium: 175mg, Phosphorus: 231mg, Potassium: 519mg

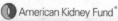

Recipe: vegan sweet potatoes n quinoa

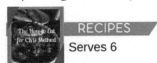

RECIPES

Serves 6

Sweet Potatoes & Quinoa

Ingredients:

1 tablespoon coconut oil (may use alternate oil)
1 cup onion, chopped
1 teaspoon sugar
1 teaspoon cumin seeds
2 teaspoons coriander seeds
1 tablespoon garlic, minced (3 cloves)
2 tablespoons ginger, minced and divided
1/2 cup roma tomatoes, diced
1 bay leaf
1/4 teaspoon ancho chili powder (or another dried red chili powder)

1/2 teaspoon kosher salt
1/2 teaspoon ground cinnamon
1/2 teaspoon pepper
1/4 teaspoon ground cardamom
1 3/4 cups water
3/4 cup dry quinoa (any color)
15 ounce can sweet potatoes, drained and diced
1/2 cup coconut milk yogurt (may use alternate yogurt)
1/4 teaspoon garam masala
3 tablespoons fresh mint, chopped
3 tablespoons dry roasted, no salt cashews, chopped

Instructions:

1. Heat the oil in a large skillet over medium heat. When hot, add the onions and sugar. Cook 8 minutes or until onions are soft and brown.
2. Add the cumin and coriander seeds and cook for 30 seconds.
3. Add the garlic and 1/2 the ginger. Cook for 30 seconds.
4. Add the tomatoes, bay leaf, chili powder, salt, cinnamon, pepper, cardamom, water, and quinoa. Stir well and bring to a boil. Reduce heat, cover, and simmer 5 minutes.
5. Add the potatoes, yogurt, masala, and the remaining ginger. Simmer 6-8 minutes or quinoa is done. (you will see little white tails coming from the quinoa).
6. Serve 1 cup per person and garnish each with 1/2 tablespoon of mint and 1/2 tablespoon of nuts.
7. Serve with naan, pita, or other bread.

Recipe tips:
- Heat this up for breakfast too!

Allergens:
Coconut, Tomato, Mint.

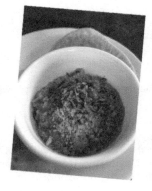

Nutrition Information:
Calculated using the NB2O system which is linked to the USDA database. Not lab tested so nutrition is not lab accurate. Calculated using ancho chili powder, coconut oil and coconut milk yogurt. Does not include bread.

Calories: 226, Fat: 7g, Sat. Fat: 3g, Trans Fat: 0g, Cholesterol: 22mg, Carbohydrates: 37g, Fiber: 4g, Sugar: 8g, Sodium: 369mg, Protein: 6g, Calcium: 94mg, Phosphorus: 174mg, Potassium: 490mg

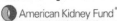

Recipe: vegan macaroni salad

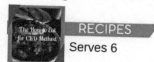
RECIPES
Serves 6

Vegan Macaroni Salad

Ingredients:

DRESSING

2 tablespoons apple cider vinegar

1 tablespoons Dijon mustard

1 tablespoon sugar

2 teaspoons fresh dill, chopped (may use 1/2 teaspoon dried)

1 teaspoon garlic powder

1/2 teaspoon pepper

1/8 teaspoon sea (kosher) salt

1/4 cup vegan sour cream

1/2 cup vegan mayonnaise

SALAD

6 ounces dry elbow macaroni or gluten free elbow macaroni noodles (3 1/4 cups cooked)

2 tablespoons jalapeno, seeds and pith removed, diced

2 full medium green onions, sliced (about 1/4 cup)

2 tablespoons fresh parsley, chopped

1 cup celery, sliced

1 cup red bell pepper, diced

Instructions:

1. Start the noodle water. Mix all dressing ingredients together until well combined. Set aside.
2. Cook noodles according to package. Drain and rinse under cold water until noodles have cooled. Set aside.
3. Combine dressing, noodles, jalapeno, green onions, parsley, celery, and bell pepper together in a bowl.
4. Chill until ready to serve. Serve a generous 1/2 cup per person.

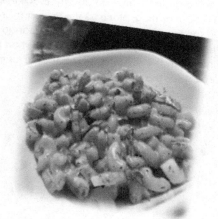

Recipe tips:

- May add 1 cup of vegan protein and double your portion to make a meal.
- If using gluten free noodles, slightly undercook them and do not combine with the rest of the ingredients until just before serving. Gluten free noodles tend to break down quickly.

Allergens:

Check Dijon, Sour Cream, Mayonnaise, and Noodles for allergens.

Nutrition Information:

Calculated using the NB2O system which is linked to the USDA database. Not lab tested so nutrition is not lab accurate. Calculated using dried dill, Hellmann's® vegan mayo and Kite-Hill® vegan sour cream. Phosphorus for nondairy sour cream is estimated.

Calories: 254, Fat: 13g, Sat. Fat: 2g, Trans Fat: 0g, Cholesterol: 0mg, Carbohydrates: 31g, Fiber: 3g, Sugar: 4g, Sodium: 240mg, Protein: 6g, Calcium: 33mg, Phosphorus: 79mg, Potassium: 198mg

Recipe created for American Kidney Fund's Kidney Kitchen®, and contributed by Linda Blaylock of CKD Culinary Consulting, ©2021 all rights reserved.

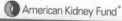 American Kidney Fund®

CKD Culinary Consulting

Recipe: mango raspberry yogurt cup

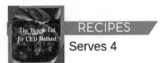

RECIPES

Serves 4

Mango-Raspberry Yogurt Cup

Ingredients:
1 cup ripe mango
4 five-ounce containers of coconut milk yogurt or about 20 ounces
1 cup raspberries
4 teaspoons fresh mint, chopped

Instructions:
1. Peel and cut the mango into small pieces, about the same size as the raspberries.
    a. Make sure your mango is ripe or the dessert will be very tangy.
    b. *To ripen the mango quickly, place in a bowl or bag with an apple overnight.
2. In a bowl or mug, place 1/2 the yogurt from one container, about 2 1/2 ounces.
3. On top layer place 1 tablespoon of mango and 1 tablespoon raspberries.
4. Place the remaining half of the yogurt on top.
5. Finish with the remaining tablespoons of mango, raspberries, and sprinkle 1 teaspoon of mint.
6. Repeat for the remaining three.

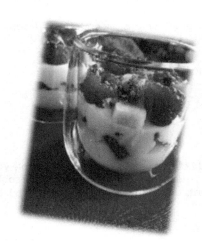

Recipe tips:
• May use other non-dairy or dairy yogurt.

Allergens:
Mango. Coconut, if using.

Nutrition Information:
Calculated using the NB2O system which is linked to the USDA database. Not lab tested so nutrition is not lab accurate. Calculated using coconut milk yogurt.

Calories: 132, Fat: 6g, Sat. Fat: 5g, Trans Fat: 0g, Cholesterol: 0mg, Carbohydrates: 22g, Fiber: 3g, Sugar: 17g, Sodium: 30mg, Protein: 1g, Calcium: 254mg, Phosphorus: 18mg, Potassium: 157mg

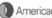

HOLIDAYS, GATHERINGS, DINING OUT, & ON-THE-GO

Here are a few tips to help you navigate these situations:

SOCIAL GATHERINGS:

- Bring a dish to share so you know there is something you can have. Inform or plan with the host.

- Know your "safe" foods and have a semi-cheat day. It is ok to have a cheat day once in a while; it is the everyday cheat days that are a problem!

- Ask about the menu plan and see what will be available to eat, then plan accordingly. Often there are fruit and vegetable trays or pasta salads.

- If having a BBQ or other event, you can ask the cook to prepare a portion without salt, sauces, etc.

- Eat before you go. If you plan to be there longer than a few hours, bring snacks or your own meal.

HOLIDAYS:

- Host. If you are the host, you can control what is on the menu. Put saltshakers out for your guests.

- If you are a guest, make your meal at home and bring it with you. Inform the host ahead of time.

- Bring a dish or two to share so you know there is something you can have. Inform or plan with the host.

- Know your "safe" foods and have a semi-cheat day.

- Ask about the menu plan and see what will be available to eat, then plan accordingly.

- Always speak with the host ahead of time. People understand dietary issues.

- Ask if you can contribute a dish or if they would rather you simply bring your own.

- Explain that you are in no way trying to offend when asking to bring a dish or if bringing a full meal for the CKD person; you are simply trying to relieve them of any worry or burden.

QUICK MEALS:

- Canned chicken or tuna to make a chicken or tuna salad sandwich.

- Purchase hard boiled eggs and/or make an egg salad sandwich.

- Fried egg & sharp cheddar sandwich.

- Oatmeal with fresh berries and cream.

- Peanut butter & jelly sandwich.

- Leftovers or meals you previously made and froze.

- Toss together some whole wheat instant couscous and chopped vegetables with a splash of oil and vinegar, and your favorite seasonings.

- Mini bagel with cream cheese. (I crazy adore a toasted bagel with guava paste/jelly and honey goat cheese. Thank me later!)

- *Look for slices of bread that are under 150mg of sodium per slice. Pepperidge Farm® makes great breads and buns that are lower in sodium and lower in additives, if any!

DINING OUT

Restaurant meals – especially at fast-casual or fast-food restaurants – can be high in sodium and over-processed foods that are filled with preservatives. Not only does this mean that eating out can be tough on your wallet, but it also means it can be tough on your kidneys.

Still, dining out is a part of our culture and you certainly can do it. However, you should try to limit the frequency of dining out or quick take out, making it a special activity rather than a routine one.

Sometimes you may find yourself in a position where the only dining options are fast-food restaurants, like when you are traveling. If you must rely on them, try to make the best choices possible from the selections available. There are some fast-food or fast-casual gems out there and you can sometimes find at least one item on the menu that you can have.

- Do your research beforehand. If the restaurant posts nutritional information for their menu items, read that information ahead of time and have a plan in place. Carry a note card (or jot it down on your phone's notes app) that lists restaurants that have menu options that fit your meal plan and the best options on their menu.

- Fast-food or fast-casual restaurants tend to have a lot of processed foods – which means they are high in sodium and potassium and/or phosphorus additives. Look for menu choices that are unseasoned and grilled or baked, have fruits and vegetables (with low to moderate potassium), and limit heavy sauces, dressing, or creams.

- Always ask for no salt or seasonings, and no sauces or dressings – or ask for them on the side. If you are eating a sandwich or hamburger, ask for no bun or substitute the bun for a lettuce wrap, if possible, or ask for no cheese.

- The "higher end" restaurants often utilize fresh ingredients and are more easily able to accommodate your requests for no salt or seasoning blends.

- Be mindful of portion sizes. Restaurants tend to serve portions that are larger than the serving size, so try eating a portion of the food and bringing the rest home.

  o If you are ordering online, it can be helpful to have one person order a meal to split with you or you may want to order a kid's entrée, side items or a la carte items to keep the portion sizes down.

- Be wary of "healthy" or vegan restaurants. Often, the sodium levels in their food are high or their meals are extremely high in potassium.

- Also, don't be fooled by the "healthy" options offered on menus. If you can, look at the sodium in those salads. They can be as bad or worse than the burgers or main items. To help, when you order a salad, choose lighter dressing options like a vinaigrette rather than a creamy ranch.

- Ask for fresh herbs on your dish, it adds beautiful pops of flavor, very little potassium, and no sodium.

- The more whole and unprocessed, the better. If you are on the go, look for things like hard boiled eggs, fruits and vegetables or salad bars. See below. (If your doctor has advised avoiding salad bars and buffets, please do so).

  o Perkins has a build a breakfast option. You can choose eggs, white bread, a side of fresh fruit and give the side of bacon or sausage to the person with you. Although we all know you are going to eat at least half a strip!

  o Subway has salads and their six-inch subs will work in a pinch.

  o Noodles & Company has a small sized buttered noodle with marinated steak. You may be able to ask them to leave off the seasoning or the marinade.

  o Red Robin has a double tavern burger with a lettuce wrap. The tavern burger patties are the safest option. Pass on all the seasonings and sauces and just top with a slice of cheese, veggies, and ketchup or mustard.

  o Five Guys soak their fresh cut fries until ready to cook. Ask for no salt on everything and have a small portion of the fries.

- If you are out with family or friends and decide to get food, request a place that has something you can eat. If possible, do a group order and have it delivered or picked up, so you can add your own salad dressings or use your own low sodium products at home.

ON THE GO:

Hardboiled eggs

Cheese stick

Small to go salad with a vinaigrette dressing

Piece of fruit

Veggie sticks

Unsalted nuts

Rice cakes

Unsalted or low sodium crackers

Mini bagel with cream cheese

Unsalted popcorn or caramel corn

Graham crackers

Jell-O or pudding cups

Vanilla wafers

Mini sandwich on bun or half a sandwich (check sodium, if low enough, or fits within your limitations, you can eat the whole thing)

Linda was the Chef for American Kidney Fund®'s Blog. A portion of this material was supplied to them on the blog. For more information, visit their site.

Thank You!

You did it!
You successfully completed this program.
I am so proud of you and look forward to continuing to help you on this journey.

This program was, and continues to be, a labor of love.
So many people, just like you, struggle to make the necessary dietary changes they need for medical reasons.
For the crazy amount of money that we must pay for health care in this country, it is truly appalling at how little we get back.
That is part of the reason for this program.

When you have a need, such as this, there should be answers, there should be guidance, there should be support, and there should be hope.
I pray that I have given you all those things.

The other reason I did this is because…
You are important, you have a purpose for being here, and there is no way we are going to let kidney disease progress without a fight.

You now have the skills and knowledge, and a ton of information for you to always come back to to get in the ring with CKD and deliver a knockout punch.

As I have mentioned many times, keep at this. It works, it gets easier.
Hey, If I can break this down into a program like this, then you know it can be done.
You know you can do it because you just did it!

You did it!

Thank you from the bottom, the top, and all sides of my heart for allowing me to aid you on this journey and to share all this knowledge and info with you.

Thank you for putting up with my silly and crazy moments and my attempts at humor and playfulness which struggle to come across in print.

Thank you for being an important part of the Facebook groups (if you had joined). Whether you are active or sit back and read everything, you are still an important part, and we always want you there.

On that note, please remain a part of the support group (if you choose to join) so you always have support when you need it. There is no way I am going to toss you out into the big, wide world on your own. You are family.

Man, could I BE any more sincere?

Some of you got that reference.

Ok. It's time to fly. Spread your wings and do so!

Knowing you have all you need, and you have your FB family supporting you and keeping you up and sailing smoothly.

Again,

Thank you.

Linda

View the video here: https://youtu.be/Dy2_64Z9pwI

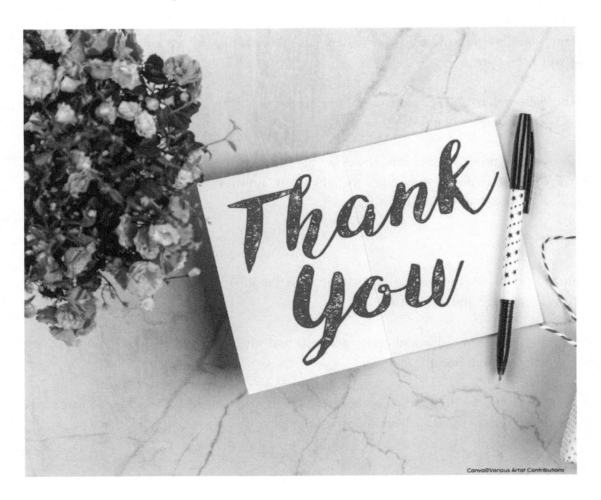

Acknowledgement

I, as always, must acknowledge my hubby and his amazing help in making this kidney diet work. Without his calculator brain and math skills, without his I.T. expertise, and more importantly, without his patience, understanding, and support, this would not be available to help others.

American Kidney Fund®, without their belief in me, without their challenges, support, and encouragement, it would have taken many, many more years to solve the kidney diet puzzle.

References

American Kidney Fund. (2022, 11 4). *Kidney Stones: Causes, Symptoms and treatment options.* Retrieved from American Kidney Fund: https://www.kidneyfund.org/all-about-kidneys/other-kidney-problems/kidney-stones

American Kidney Fund. (n.d.). *Polycistic Kidney Disease (PKD) symptoms, treatments & causes.* Retrieved from American Kidney Fund: https://www.kidneyfund.org/all-about-kidneys/types-kidney-diseases/polycystic-kidney-disease

American Kidney Fund. (n.d.). *Pruritus.* Retrieved from American Kidney Fund: https://www.kidneyfund.org/living-kidney-disease/health-problems-caused-kidney-disease/pruritus-itchy-skin

Bhandari S, K. Z. (Am J Nephrol 2022;53:32–40). *Causes of Death in End-Stage Kidney Disease: Comparison between the United States Renal Data System and a Large Integrated Health Care System.* Retrieved from Karger: https://www.karger.com/Article/FullText/520466#

Cleaveland Clinic. (n.d.). *Hyperoxaluria.* Retrieved from Cleaveland Clinic: https://my.clevelandclinic.org/health/diseases/21117-hyperoxaluria

Mayo Clinic. (n.d.). *Hemodialysis.* Retrieved from Mayo Clinic: https://www.mayoclinic.org/diseases-conditions/end-stage-renal-disease/multimedia/hemodialysis/vid-20231485

Mayo Clinic. (n.d.). *Peritoneal dialysis.* Retrieved from Mayo Clinic: https://www.mayoclinic.org/tests-procedures/peritoneal-dialysis/about/pac-20384725

National Institute of Health. (n.d.). *Autosomal recessive polycystic kidney disease.* Retrieved from NHS: https://www.nhs.uk/conditions/autosomal-recessive-polycystic-kidney-disease-arpkd/#:~:text=Autosomal%20recessive%20polycystic%20kidney%20disease%20(ARPKD)%20is%20a%20rare%20inherited,time%2C%20these%20organs%20may%20fail.

National Kidney Foundation. (n.d.). *Recommendations for Implementing the CKD-EPI 2021 Race-Free eGFR Calculation: Guidelines for Clinical Laboratories.* Retrieved from National Kidney Foundation: https://www.kidney.org/content/national-kidney-foundation-laboratory-engagement-working-group-recommendations-implementing

Shaikh H, H. M. (2023, 2 24). *Anemia of Chronic Renal Disease.* Retrieved from National Library of Medicine: https://www.ncbi.nlm.nih.gov/books/NBK539871/

U.S. Food & Drug Administration. (2022, Feb. 25). *Daily Value on the New Nutrition and Supplement Facts Labels.* Retrieved from FDA: https://www.fda.gov/food/new-nutrition-facts-label/daily-value-new-nutrition-and-supplement-facts-labels

Various. (n.d.). *Photos and Fonts.* Canva.

About The Author

Linda is the Owner of CKD Culinary Consulting™ and is the creator and owner of The How to Eat for CKD Method™ program.

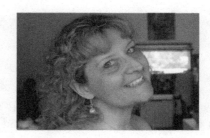

She is a chef honors graduate of Escoffier School of Culinary Arts®, an ISSA® Certified Nutritionist, a certified kidney health coach, and a caregiver to her husband who has stage 3 kidney disease.

She was a culinary consultant for American Kidney Fund®, and many of her recipes are available on their Kidney Kitchen® website; she was also the chef contributing educational content to their blog. Linda has done informational webinars and cooking demonstrations for American Kidney Fund® and National Kidney Foundation®. She has been in Culinary Entrepreneurs® magazine and has worked with dieticians to further client's kidney diet success and help make the transition into CKD eating an easy and fully informed one.

She enjoys exploring unfamiliar cuisines and adapting them, as well as finding historical recipes to CKD-ify and improve.

Before meeting her (second) husband, she was a single mother with three (adorable and cute) young children. Living on a budget, being creative, and relying on easy to find ingredients is her specialty.

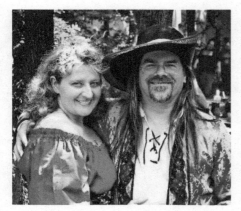

When her husband received his diagnosis, she was graduating college for business management and prepping a business plan to open a clinic with friends.

The demands of trying to figure out how to "save" her husband were immense. She had to (heartbreakingly) go to the group and tell them she was out. She felt she needed to put 100% of her time into solving the CKD puzzle.

So, within a week of graduating, she turned around and went to culinary school, then followed that with more for nutrition. The entire time, she was devoted to finding the answers and applying all she was learning into how it fit best with CKD.

It took her five years, but thankfully she had been blessed with the ability to focus solely on it, and to be in the right place, at the right time, with the right education, opportunities, and the right circumstances to find every vital answer.

After two years of painstakingly assembling the program, she brought it forward to help others. Her husband's lab numbers have remained stable all these years, although, his pants size did go up from all the amazingly tasty foods.

She lives in Minneapolis with her pet bearded dragons, her chubby cat, Butters Karen (some of you will get that reference), and her husband. When she isn't creating recipes, overseeing her program and groups, filling orders, researching new products, creating, or perfecting recipes, or keeping up with the latest CKD news, supporting her clients, or working on her cookbooks ...

You will find her gathering with family as often as possible, playing a Pathfinder® card game with her husband and/or friends, frequenting Renaissance Fairs, reading about Native American or Viking history, physics, philosophy, historical cooking, or binge watching El Reencuentro Menudo videos online, or snuggling her dragons while watching historical dramas, Miranda, Living Single, & Gilmore Girls reruns, Ghost Adventures, or Guy's Grocery Games with her husband.

We know... she's a weird one!

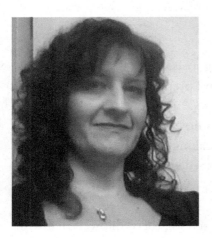

A percentage of proceeds from sales are donated to American Kidney Fund®, so they may further help those with kidney disease that are in need.

Made in the USA
Coppell, TX
04 June 2023

17661155R00118